Dizziness

A Practical Approach to Diagnosis and Management

Second Edition

Dizziness

A Practical Approach to Diagnosis and Management

Second Edition

Adolfo Bronstein
Clinical Professor, Neuro-otology Unit, Division of Brain Sciences, Imperial College London, UK

Thomas Lempert
Professor, Charité University Hospital and Department of Neurology, Schlosspark-Klinik, Berlin, Germany

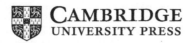
CAMBRIDGE
UNIVERSITY PRESS

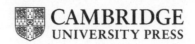

Shaftesbury Road, Cambridge CB2 8EA, United Kingdom

One Liberty Plaza, 20th Floor, New York, NY 10006, USA

477 Williamstown Road, Port Melbourne, VIC 3207, Australia

314–321, 3rd Floor, Plot 3, Splendor Forum, Jasola District Centre,
New Delhi – 110025, India

103 Penang Road, #05–06/07, Visioncrest Commercial, Singapore 238467

Cambridge University Press is part of a Cambridge University Press & Assessment,
a department of the University of Cambridge.

We share the University's mission to contribute to society through the pursuit of
education, learning and research at the highest international levels of excellence.

www.cambridge.org
Information on this title: www.cambridge.org/9781107663909

First published 2007
Second edition 2017 (version 5, August 2023)

Printed in Great Britain by Ashford Colour Press Ltd.

A catalogue record for this publication is available from the British Library

Library of Congress Cataloging-in-Publication Data
Names: Bronstein, Adolfo M., author. | Lempert, Thomas, author.
Title: Dizziness : a practical approach to diagnosis and management / Adolfo
Bronstein, Thomas Lempert.
Description: Second edition. | Cambridge ; New York : Cambridge University
Press, 2017. | Includes bibliographical references and index.
Identifiers: LCCN 2016011753| ISBN 9781316621578 (paperback : alk.
paper) | ISBN 9781107663909 (mixed media)
Subjects: | MESH: Dizziness–diagnosis | Dizziness–therapy | Vertigo–
diagnosis | Vertigo–therapy
Classification: LCC RB150.V4 | NLM WL 340 | DDC 616.8/41–dc23 LC
record available at http://lccn.loc.gov/2016011753

ISBN 978-1-107-66390-9 Mixed media product
ISBN 978-1-316-62157-8 Paperback
ISBN 978-1-316-75646-1 Cambridge Core

Additional resources for this publication at www.cambridge.org/
9781107663909

....

Contents

Tables

Video clips on accompanying website

Introduction: how to use this book

Don't read this book — from cover to cover! This book has been written for the non-expert doctor who sees dizzy patients and who needs quick guidance to differential diagnosis and treatment. Conventional books are not always helpful in this situation as they are disease-oriented, and only after reading them from A to Z might you guess what your actual patient's problem is. This book is different in taking a symptom-oriented approach.

The book starts with two introductory chapters which deal with the essential anatomy and functions of the vestibular system and with the clinical assessment of the dizzy patient. These chapters are required reading as they prepare the ground for working with dizzy patients. From there on, you can turn directly to one of the problem-oriented chapters whenever you need to solve a particular dizziness problem. The clinical chapters are entitled according to common and easily identifiable clinical situations such as positional vertigo or recurrent dizziness. Each clinical chapter begins with a table for differential diagnosis with key features of the relevant disorders, followed by a concise text organised in the same sequence as the opening table. Numerous other tables facilitate the differential diagnosis. Common disorders are explained in detail, rarities are only briefly touched on. At the end of each of the clinical chapters you will find a section entitled 'What to do if you don't have a clue' that gives you some rescue ideas to manage impossible clinical situations.

The final chapter, 'Treatment of the dizzy patient', explains general aspects of treatment such as the use of vestibular sedatives and the principles of vestibular rehabilitation which are common to various disorders. The more specific aspects of treatment are dealt with in the dedicated chapters. The accompanying website material shows the clinical examination, the diagnostic and therapeutic positioning manoeuvres for benign paroxysmal positional vertigo, and exercises for vestibular rehabilitation, as well as examples of common clinical findings. Each chapter refers you to the corresponding video clips on the website, although you may prefer to see them all in one go by way of a 'hands on' introduction on how to deal with a dizzy patient.

The world of dizziness has changed completely in the last two decades, as new treatable syndromes have been identified, such as vestibular migraine, the variants of benign paroxysmal positional vertigo, and psychiatric causes of dizziness. We hope that this book will stimulate your interest in vertigo and balance disorders and that it will make you feel optimistic when facing your next dizzy patient.

Essential anatomy and functions of the balance system

Introduction

If you are reading this book you are almost certainly a busy clinician. We understand your apprehension at having to go back and review some basic anatomy and physiology concepts. All we can say is that everything you will see in this chapter will have a direct application in the diagnosis and management of your dizzy patient. One other preliminary comment: immediately after the three main headings in this chapter you will find *brief summaries* on pages 2, 11 and 15. You can read these summaries straight away, if you are conversant with the subject or wish to know what the content of this chapter is – but this may feel heavy going. Alternatively, you can come back to each of the summaries once you have read the whole section, to consolidate what you have learnt.

Normal balance is the consequence of continuous interaction between vestibular, proprioceptive and visual mechanisms, which in turn are integrated and modulated by all levels of the central nervous system (CNS). A lesion or dysfunction in any of these mechanisms can create balance problems per se or interfere with the recovery of otherwise straightforward vestibular disorders. For instance, a patient with an acute viral infection of the vestibular nerve (vestibular neuritis), even if it causes permanent unilateral absence of vestibular function, could recover quickly if the patient is a young, fit person. The same vestibular lesion can lead to permanent balance symptoms in an elderly person with age-related dysfunction of the visual, proprioceptive or central nervous systems.

Anatomy and physiology of the vestibular system

Summary

- The labyrinth is just one component in the balance system. However, most causes of dizziness are inner-ear problems.
- The semicircular canals (horizontal, anterior and posterior) sense angular head acceleration. The otoliths (utricle and saccule) sense linear head acceleration, including gravity.
- Each ear has three canals and two otoliths. Note that most vestibular tests examine only the horizontal canal, one-fifth of the vestibular labyrinth.
- The superior vestibular nerve contains afferents from the superior and horizontal canals and from the utricle. The inferior vestibular nerve carries the fibres from the inferior (posterior) canal and the saccule. This organisation explains why vestibular neuritis patients can have loss of horizontal canal function and posterior canal BPPV (benign paroxysmal positional vertigo).

- The vascular supply approximately follows the neural innervation – this is why vascular lesions can involve preferentially the cochlea or the vestibule. However, except when there is selective terminal branch arterial involvement, both organs (and the brainstem) are equally involved.
- Background discharge in the vestibular nerve (vestibular tone or tonus) explains why a unilateral vestibular lesion produces vertigo even in the absence of any head movements. It also explains why the remaining labyrinth can signal head movements in all directions: movements in the 'on' direction increase background discharge whereas movements in the 'off' direction reduce the background discharge.

Most readers of this book will be medical graduates and will have studied anatomy and physiology as separate subjects. Here we will try to combine these disciplines, and whenever possible, pathology as well, because an integrated approach will be more useful for clinicians.

The actual symptoms (dizziness, vertigo, imbalance; see Chapter 2) in patients with various vestibular disorders are often similar. In many cases even the traditional distinction between vertigo and dizziness does not apply. The diagnosis often therefore depends on additional symptoms, which in many cases are due to extension of the causative lesion into neighbouring structures. For this reason it is important to know not only vestibular anatomy but also what structures are in the vicinity of vestibular structures or pathways.

The labyrinth consists of the bony labyrinth in the petrous section of the temporal bone and the membranous labyrinth contained therein. The sensory epithelium, which transduces sound (cochlear) and head motion (vestibular), is located within the membranous labyrinth. The membranous labyrinth contains the endolymphatic fluid which bathes the sensory epithelium; the perilymph is the fluid present between the bony and membranous labyrinths. The vestibular (or posterior) labyrinth comprises organs specialised to transduce angular acceleration, the semicircular canals, and organs specialised to transduce linear and gravitational acceleration, the otolith organs.

Semicircular canals

There are three semicircular canals on each side, one horizontal and two vertical. They are positioned approximately orthogonally and so they can sense angular movements in any plane and direction (Figure 1.1). These semicircular canal planes are complementary on each side of the head so that head movements are complementarily signalled by a pair of functionally coplanar canals:

- The horizontal (or lateral) canals sense horizontal head rotation ('no–no movements').
- Diagonal or oblique head movements (e.g. first turn your head horizontally 45° to the right and then bend your neck up and down) are signalled by the combination of an anterior (or superior) canal on one side and a posterior (or inferior) canal on the other. In this example, the oscillation indicated will be sensed by the left anterior and right posterior canals (Figure 1.1).
- A purely sagittal head-down movement ('yes–yes movements') stimulates both anterior canals and inhibits both posterior canals; head-up movements do the opposite.
- A roll head movement, such as bringing the right ear down towards the right shoulder, stimulates both anterior and posterior canals on the right, and inhibits both vertical canals on the opposite side.

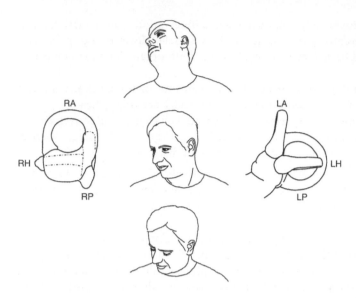

Figure 1.1 Orientation of semi-circular canals. The figure highlights pairs of canals that are activated by an oblique head movement. If you oscillate your head up and down, while your head is turned some 45 degrees to the right, the oscillatory movement is detected by the left anterior (superior) canal and the right posterior (inferior) canal (LA and RP, respectively – the LARP plane). If you were to turn the head 45 degrees to the left and repeat the up–down movement, you would be stimulating the right anterior and left posterior canal – the RALP plane.

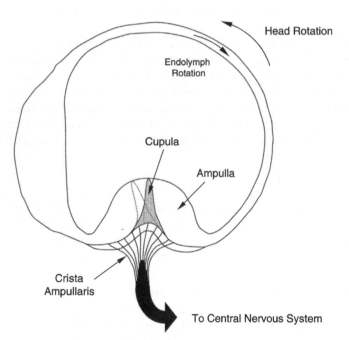

Figure 1.2 Semicircular canal activation. As the skull rotates in one direction the endolymph is relatively displaced in the opposite. This endolymph motion exerts pressure on the cupula which thus activates the sensory epithelium. During a long-duration rotation (> 30 s) there is no longer relative endolymph displacement with respect to the head and thus canal stimulation gradually ceases.

The mechanism of activation of a semicircular canal is shown in Figure 1.2. Each canal has an open end, which communicates freely with the vestibule, and an enlarged or ampular end, where the sensory epithelium, the cupula, is housed. It is important to remember that each canal has an open and a closed (cupular) end – particle repositioning treatments for benign paroxysmal positional vertigo (BPPV) rely on you moving the patient's head appropriately so that intracanalicular particles leave the canal through the open end.

The cupula is a gelatinous conglomerate of sensory hair cells – it is the bending of the cupula, and therefore of the hair or cilia, that generates bioelectrical activity and action potentials down the vestibular nerve. What makes the cupula bend is the pressure exerted by the endolymph during head rotation. As Figure 1.2 shows, head rotation to the left produces relative motion of the endolymph fluid in the opposite direction, which thus deflects the cupula.

In summary, the CNS knows *in what plane* the head has rotated by the pattern of activation of the various individual canals. The CNS knows *how fast* the head has rotated by the frequency rate of the action potentials in the vestibular nerve, which is in turn dependent on the magnitude of the endolymph-induced cupular deflection.

Vestibular tone or tonus

The concept of vestibular tonus is important as it has fairly immediate clinical significance. Essentially the term tonus is used because, even in the absence of any rotation, semicircular canal afferents in the vestibular nerve show a resting or 'tonic' discharge. Each canal has an angular direction in which cupular deflection increases the discharge in the vestibular nerve (the 'on' direction), and the opposite 'off' direction which decreases neural activity in canal afferents. The orientation of the ciliae is such that horizontal head acceleration to the right is 'on' for the right horizontal canal and 'off' for the left one. The brain knows that the head is turning because on one side neural activity increases whilst it decreases on the other.

The practical implications include the following:

1. The existence of a resting vestibular tone explains why a patient with unilateral hypofunction experiences vertigo even without making any head movement. The CNS detects a difference in discharge rate between the two sides and 'assumes' that the head is rotating.

2. Even in the presence of a total and permanent unilateral semicircular canal lesion, the brain is capable of sensing angular movements in all directions. The remaining labyrinth can signal both directions of motion due to the on–off arrangement. This bidirectional capacity of a single canal provides the basis for the phenomenon of *vestibular compensation* which underlies recovery of function and symptoms in patients with unilateral vestibular lesions.

Short and long rotations

How the semicircular canals work during brief and long rotations also has to be understood as there are clinical implications here too.

Brisk brief rotations

The on–off arrangement described above is not perfectly symmetrical. During accelerations in the 'on' direction, canal afferents have almost no saturation; vestibular nerve activity increases linearly with the velocity of the rotation. Rotations in the 'off' direction, however, do reach a saturation point as the decrease in vestibular nerve activity can reach down only to zero – there is not such a thing as a negative discharge rate.

A clinical consequence is that during a very fast acceleration towards the side of a lesion, angular velocity will not be faithfully transduced by the remaining labyrinth as it is working in the 'off' direction. Patients can therefore report symptoms such as unsteadiness, dizziness or oscillopsia during fast head movements towards the lesion side.

This phenomenon also provides the basis of an important clinical finding, the positive 'head-impulse' or 'head-thrust' sign (see page 36). Essentially, during a fast head rotation towards the side of the lesion the vestibularly driven compensatory eye movement is insufficient. Instead of a smooth compensatory eye movement, the clinician observes a refixation saccade, indicative of a hypoactive labyrinth on the side of the head turn. This will become clearer later under 'Vestibulo-ocular reflex'.

Long-duration rotations

Cupular deflection during rotations occurs thanks to the endolymph inertia. Think of a soup (the endolymph) in a bowl (your skull). If you suddenly turn the bowl, the bowl moves but the soup doesn't. This relative motion between the endolymph and the semicircular canal is what makes the cupula bend. This difference will be maximal at the onset of movement, i.e. if you place the bowl on a turntable, after a while the bowl and the soup will be turning at the same speed. For this reason – namely that cupular deflection will be maximal at the onset or accelerative phase of movement – one has to think of the canals as angular accelerometers, which measure the change in velocity rather than velocity itself.

As in the culinary example given, if head rotation continues at constant speed there will be a point where skull and endolymph rotate at the same speed (i.e. there is no relative motion between endolymph and semicircular canal). During prolonged rotations, then, cupular deflection, and hence dynamic vestibular input, progressively decays and eventually stops altogether after 15–20 seconds into constant rotation. But then, if the body stops rotating, the inertia of the endolymph will deflect the cupula in the reverse direction – this explains why you feel as if you are turning when you stop a prolonged rotation such as stepping off a merry-go-round or after rolling downhill.

This is the basis of the 'stopping' response test during vestibular testing with rotatory Baranyi chairs. You can try the following experiment. Seat somebody on an office swivel chair, turn him round for 20–30 seconds and then stop him quite suddenly. The subject will feel vertiginous and, if you look at his eyes carefully, you will see a jerky beating of the eyes called *vestibular nystagmus*. If you time the duration of the nystagmus when stopping from right versus left rotation, you will have an indication of the degree of symmetry in vestibular activity – the essence of all vestibular tests.

Otolith system

The otoliths sense head linear acceleration. Since gravity is linear acceleration, the otoliths also sense head tilt with respect to the gravity vector. There are two sets of otolith organs per side, the utricle and the saccule. These are shown schematically in Figure 1.3.

What makes the otolithic hair cells sensitive to linear acceleration is the fact that the gelatinous membrane embedding the ciliae of the hair cells is loaded with heavy calcium crystals called otoconia. As the head accelerates, the heavy otolith membrane is 'left behind', thus deflecting hair cells and generating action potentials in the vestibular afferents. The approximately horizontal orientation of the utricles makes them sensitive to linear accelerations in the horizontal plane. The sacculi are placed approximately in a parasagittal orientation and are therefore sensitive to linear accelerations occurring in the sagittal plane. It is apparent that the otolith organs also have some sensitivity to sound and this feature has some clinical relevance as new laboratory tests called VEMPs (vestibular-evoked myogenic potentials) use loud sounds, usually clicks, to activate them.

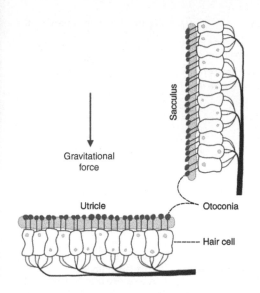

Figure 1.3 Otolith organs. Note the gelatinous membrane loaded with otoconia (calcium particles). In the normal upright position the utricle lies approximately horizontal and the sacculus approximately vertical. In this position the force of gravity (arrow) will predominantly deflect the hair cells in the saccular organs. Note that linear head acceleration upwards will have the same effect.

It is important to bear in mind that normal head movements combine linear and angular accelerations in any plane and direction. The exquisite arrangement of four otolith organs and six semicircular canals is capable of transducing any such complex movements. At this point, we would like to remind readers that most of the traditional tests of vestibular function concentrate on horizontal semicircular canal function (caloric and rotational tests), namely 20% of the vestibular system! This is no doubt one of the reasons why so many patients have vestibular symptoms but normal vestibular function tests.

Innervation and blood supply of the labyrinth

Each of the semicircular canals and otolith organs receives afferent innervation (singular nerves) from the vestibular nerve (Figure 1.4). Before reaching the Scarpa ganglion (where the neuronal body of these afferents is) the singular nerves are grouped into an inferior and a superior component. The superior vestibular nerve contains the fibres from the superior (anterior) and horizontal canals and from the utricle. The inferior vestibular nerve carries the fibres from the inferior (posterior) canal and the saccule. The vestibular nerve comprises the axons of the Scarpa ganglion neurons, which then enter the porus of the internal acoustic meatus, posteriorly to the cochlear nerve, forming the vestibulo-cochlear nerve or VIII cranial nerve.

This anatomical distribution explains a few clinical points. For instance, viral vestibular neuritis or 'neuronitis' usually involves the superior vestibular nerve only. The loss of horizontal canal function explains the caloric canal paresis (see pages 36, 47 and 56). The utricular involvement can lead to degeneration of the otoconia and to the release of calcium crystals into the vestibule, from where they can fall into the lumen of the posterior semicircular canal. This is why some patients develop positional vertigo after an episode of vestibular neuritis: the spared inferior vestibular nerve and posterior canal are able to sense the abnormal endolymph currents created by the intraluminal otoconia (see Figure 5.1).

Arterial irrigation to the labyrinth comes from the internal auditory artery, which is usually a branch of the anterior inferior cerebellar artery (AICA) or, less frequently, of the basilar artery. The internal auditory artery gives off a branch called the anterior vestibular

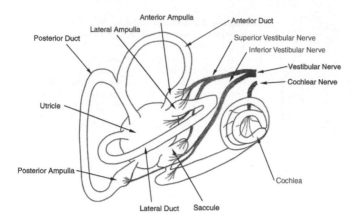

Anterior Ampulla
Lateral Ampulla
Posterior Duct
Anterior Duct
Superior Vestibular Nerve
Inferior Vestibular Nerve
Vestibular Nerve
Cochlear Nerve
Utricle
Posterior Ampulla
Cochlea
Lateral Duct   Saccule

Figure 1.4 Innervation of the labyrinth. The two divisions of the vestibular nerve, the superior and inferior vestibular nerve, are shown.

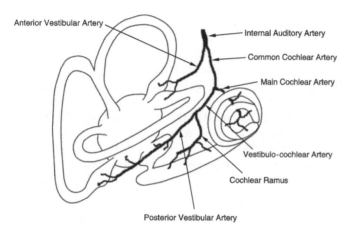

Anterior Vestibular Artery
Internal Auditory Artery
Common Cochlear Artery
Main Cochlear Artery
Vestibulo-cochlear Artery
Cochlear Ramus
Posterior Vestibular Artery

Figure 1.5 Arterial blood supply to the labyrinth. The internal auditory artery is a branch of the anterior inferior cerebellar artery, or AICA (not shown). The structures irrigated by the anterior vestibular artery correspond to those innervated by the superior vestibular nerve (Figure 1.4), principally the anterior and horizontal semicircular canals.

artery, which irrigates the anterior and horizontal canals and the utricle (the same structures innervated by the superior vestibular nerve) (Figure 1.5). The internal auditory artery continues as the common cochlear artery and it divides into two terminal arteries: (a) the vestibulo-cochlear artery, irrigating the inferior (posterior) canal, the sacculus (just what the inferior vestibular nerve innervates) and the basal turn of the cochlea, and (b) the main cochlear artery serving the bulk of the cochlea.

It can be seen that, as in other body regions, neural and vascular supply converge considerably. Accordingly, an acute selective lesion of the anterior/horizontal canals, sparing hearing, could be equally produced by vascular ischaemia of the anterior vestibular artery or neuritis of the superior vestibular nerve (as in vestibular neuritis).

Another applied concept explains the 'AICA syndrome', which combines unilateral deafness, canal paresis and cerebellar dysfunction, all on the same side. This is due to the fact that the internal auditory artery usually branches off the anterior inferior cerebellar artery. In view of the known anatomy, we would argue that the likelihood should be very small of recurrent vertigo in isolation (i.e. no cochlear or cerebellar–brainstem–occipital lobe symptoms) being due to vertebrobasilar ischaemia or a transient ischaemic attack (TIA). Based on this anatomical fact, clinicians should refrain from overdiagnosing

Table 1.1 Central vestibular projections and their symptoms

Projections	Symptoms
Vestibulo-cortical	Vertigo
Vestibulo-ocular	Nystagmus
Vestibulo-spinal	Unsteadiness
Vestibulo-autonomic-limbic	Nausea, sweating, anxiety

Table 1.2 Localisation and structures

Neighbouring structures as the basis of topographic diagnosis	
Inner ear/temporal bone	Cochlea and cochlear nerve
Internal auditory meatus	Cranial nerves V, VI, VII and cochlear nerve
Brainstem	Cranial nerves III, IV, V, VI, VII, IX, X and cerebellum

'vascular vertigo' due to 'vertebro-basilar insufficiency' when there are no accompanying auditory or CNS symptoms.

Central pathways

The vestibular pathway starts with the primary vestibular neurons in Scarpa's (vestibular) ganglion in the temporal bone. These neurons project on to the secondary vestibular neurons in the vestibular nuclei of the brainstem. From here axons project to (a) thalamo-cortical structures, (b) oculomotor nuclei via the medial longitudinal fasciculus (MLF), (c) the spinal cord, (d) the cerebellum and (e) autonomic medullary centres (Figure 1.6). This is a perfect example of anatomic–clinical correlation because these projections explain why patients with vestibular lesions have, respectively, (a) a conscious illusion of spinning (vertigo), (b) nystagmus, (c) lateropulsion, (d) gait ataxia, and (e) autonomic symptoms such as nausea, vomiting and sweating (Table 1.1).

Topographical diagnosis

There are two important aspects of clinically applied anatomy. One is the function that is lost when a structure or pathway is damaged. The other is the structures that are near a pathway of interest; in our case, what is near the vestibular pathway at various anatomical regions. The first point is easy for us – vestibular lesions at all levels, from the ear to the cortex, will produce dizziness, vertigo or imbalance. For the second point, we need to remember the neighbouring structures and this is the basis of topographical diagnosis. Within the temporal bone, these are the organ of Corti and the cochlear nerve; as we leave the internal auditory meatus, the V, VI and VII cranial nerves are neighbours of the vestibulo-cochlear (VIII) nerve (Table 1.2).

Vestibular and cochlear pathways separate soon after entering the brainstem at the pontomedullary junction, as they proceed to their respective vestibular (medial) and cochlear (lateral) nuclei. This explains two facts:

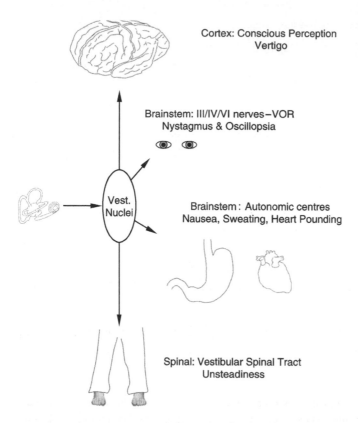

Cortex: Conscious Perception
Vertigo

Brainstem: III/IV/VI nerves–VOR
Nystagmus & Oscillopsia

Vest.
Nuclei

Brainstem: Autonomic centres
Nausea, Sweating, Heart Pounding

Spinal: Vestibular Spinal Tract
Unsteadiness

Figure 1.6 Central projections of the vestibular nerve, explaining the symptoms in acute vestibular disorders: vertigo (cortex), nystagmus and oscillopsia (ocular motor nerves), unsteadiness (vestibulospinal tracts) and autonomic symptoms. VOR: vestibulo-ocular reflex.

- There is a high frequency of associated ipsilateral hearing problems in labyrinthine, temporal-bone and extra-axial brainstem pathology.
- There is a rarity of clinically obvious hearing problems in central vestibular disorders. This is due not only to the separation of vestibular and cochlear pathways in the CNS but also to the multiple crossings and bilateral representation of central auditory pathways.

Recall from anatomy lessons that the brainstem is a small structure comprising many vital nuclei and pathways. And yet, within this tightly packed formation, vestibular representation is quite large (no doubt indicating the evolutionary weight placed on balance function). For these reasons, almost any structure in the brainstem is a 'neighbour' to the central vestibular system, and this explains why vestibular symptoms and signs are so common in brainstem lesions. In the vicinity of vestibular pathways are cranial nerve structures accounting for symptoms of diplopia (III, IV, VI), facial numbness (V) or weakness (VII), and swallowing or speech difficulties (IX, X) (Figure 1.7). The strong functional interaction between the vestibular and cerebellar systems explains the presence of vertigo in cerebellar lesions. Reciprocally, there is frequently cerebellar ataxia in central vestibular lesions, owing to the anatomical closeness of vestibular structures and the three cerebellar peduncles.

- Long-tract symptoms such as hemianaesthesia and hemiparesis are relatively less common in central vestibular disorders than cerebellar/cranial nerves ones. This is due to the fact that the cortico-spinal (pyramidal) and somatosensory (medial lemniscus) pathways are in the ventral (anterior) segment, whereas vestibular pathways are located in the dorsal tegmentum of the brainstem, towards the floor of the IV ventricle (Figure 1.7).

(A)

(B)

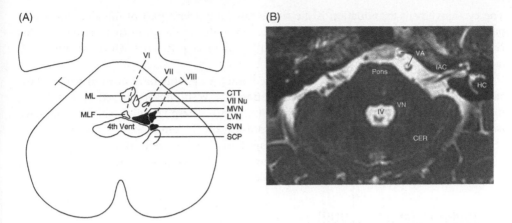

Figure 1.7 Vestibular 'neighbours' in the brainstem (lower pontine level). A: The lateral (L), medial (M) and superior (S) vestibular nucleus (VN) at the floor of the fourth ventricle. The sixth (VI) nerve and the medial longitudinal fascicle (MLF) are responsible for visual symptoms, such as diplopia. The seventh (VII) nerve and fifth (not shown), are responsible for facial weakness and numbness respectively. Involvement of the central tegmental tract (CTT) and superior cerebellar peduncle (SCP) can lead to ataxia. The medial lemniscus (ML) carries somatic sensation of the contralateral side of the body, giving rise to symptoms of tingling or numbness (modified from Lopez et al., 1992). B: MRI at the corresponding level (CISS sequence). Relevant structures include the internal auditory canal (IAC) containing the vestibulo-cochlear and facial nerve, vertebral arteries (VA), horizontal canal (HC), vestibular nuclei (VN), cerebellum (CER) and fourth ventricle (IV).

At a cortical level, it is debated whether there are any exclusive vestibular areas, as opposed to multisensory areas engaged in spatial orientation, and this may explain the rarity of vertigo in cortical lesions. Rotational vertigo can be evoked by electrical stimulation or lesions in the insular cortex, sometimes referred to as the parieto-insular vestibular cortex (PIVC).

Eye movements

Summary

- We consider two types of eye movement:
    - gaze stabilising (slow-phase movements): VOR (vestibulo-ocular reflex) and smooth pursuit;
    - gaze transferring (fast-phase movements): saccades and quick nystagmic phases.
- The function of the VOR is to stabilise the eyes in space during head movements. Suspect a VOR problem when vision is 'wobbly' during head movements.
- VOR suppression is a pursuit-mediated mechanism that suppresses the VOR when you want to foveate an object that rotates with you (e.g. like looking at your wristwatch while you turn a corner).
- Pursuit allows fixation, and thus clear vision, of slowly moving objects.
- Saccades are fast eye movements that allow you to fixate on different objects.
- Rules of thumb:
    - peripheral vestibular disorders produce abnormal VOR but spare other eye movements;
    - central disorders may produce abnormal pursuit, VOR suppression and saccades with or without VOR problems.

The eye-movement examination is the single most important part of the assessment of a patient with a balance disorder. Its overall value is only second to history-taking. For this reason it is essential to understand a few physiological principles which, in turn, will facilitate the understanding of clinical signs.

The eyes move in order to see better. Oculomotor systems have evolved which allow stabilisation of our eyes both during self-motion (the vestibulo-ocular reflex) and during movements of visual objects (smooth-pursuit system). These visually stabilising mechanisms are called *slow-phase* mechanisms. In contrast, quick components of nystagmus and saccades, which take the eyes from one object to another (refixations), are *fast-phase* mediated. These systems have different anatomical and physiological bases and, therefore, different localisation value for clinical purposes.

Vestibulo-ocular reflex (VOR)

The diagnosis of the dizzy patient relies so much on the clinical, and sometimes laboratory, assessment of the VOR that a small introductory section on this reflex is needed. The VOR is an old and simple reflex with only three synapses between the ear and the eye; one between the VIII-nerve fibres and the vestibular nuclei, one between the vestibular nuclei fibres and the oculomotor nuclei (III, IV or VI), and one neuromuscular synapse between the oculomotor nuclei and the extra-ocular eye muscles. This reduced neuronal arrangement guarantees fast and efficient ear-to-eye transmission.

The function of the VOR is to stabilise the eyes in space during head movements. The eye has often been compared to a camera; but have you ever wondered how come that, in order to take a clear picture we have to hold the camera very still whereas we always see clearly despite our head moving about all the time? The answer is that we have a VOR but the camera does not.

The way the VOR works is by generating eye movements of the same speed, but opposite in direction, to head movements. If you oscillate your head up and down at different velocities whilst looking at an object in front of you, you will be able to continue to see the object selected clearly. Your semicircular canals transduce the velocity of your head movement accurately and converts it into a neural impulse that in turn drives the eyes at the required speed. However, in a patient with acute loss of vestibular function on one side, when the head (nose) turns towards the lesion this process is faulty and the eye movement generated is of insufficient speed. The subjective consequence will be blurred or 'wobbly' vision (oscillopsia). An attentive observer (you!) looking at this patient's eyes will notice that during a fast horizontal head turn in the direction of the *healthy labyrinth* the eyes remain perfectly on target. When turning the head fast in the opposite direction (towards the *damaged labyrinth*) the eyes will need a couple of 'catch-up' saccades to be able to refixate the visual object selected. This indicates that the horizontal semicircular canal on this side is at fault. This is the basis of the clinical 'head-thrust' or 'head-impulse' test (see page 36).

If a patient shows 'catch-up' saccades during head turns to both right and left he almost certainly has a severe bilateral vestibular lesion. As a consequence his vision will be wobbly (oscillopsia) every time he moves, for instance when he walks, runs or rides in a car. Further details on how to examine the VOR clinically can be found on pages 36 and 37 (Figures 2.2 and 2.3).

One of the characteristics of the VOR is that its optimum working range is at high frequencies and fast velocities of head motion. This means that the VOR is specialised in stabilising the eyes during fast/high-frequency movements of the head, in sharp contrast to visuomotor mechanisms such as pursuit or optokinetic eye movements which only work at relatively slow movements of the visual stimulus. Try this simple experiment. Hold a book at arms' length, keep it still and move your head continuously from side to side ('no–no–no–no'), pretty fast, whilst attempting to read. You should be able to carry on reading quite well. Now keep the head still and try to move the book at a similar rate (frequency and amplitude) whilst attempting to read. In this case you are likely to have great difficulty in reading because you are using pursuit rather than VOR to stabilise gaze on the text. The many synapses and long delays inherent to the visual and visuomotor systems, in contrast to the fast VOR transduction and transmission, make them unsuitable for image stabilisation at fast frequencies and velocities.

During large-amplitude head movements, say more than 45°, eye position in the orbit has to be reset and this is brought about by quick phases. The alternating succession of slow (stabilising) and quick (resetting) phases during large-angle rotations is what produces physiological vestibular nystagmus. If you now stand up in the middle of the room and turn round fully two or three times you will be able to see fairly clearly features all around the room. The slow phase of the VOR is what allows the fairly stable and clear vision. The fast resetting phases allow your eyes to switch from one visual target to another. This sequence also stops extreme eye-in-orbit deviations happening and provides the basis for a reflex visual scanning mechanism, as you should have noticed if you did do the suggested experiment.

These resetting quick phases are essentially small involuntary saccades. During normal head movements there is a synergy between vestibular (VOR) and visual (pursuit, optokinetic) mechanisms. However, quite often there is conflict or antagonism between vestibular and visuomotor mechanisms, as we shall see next under 'VOR suppression'.

VOR suppression

Imagine yourself walking round a corner. As you walk round, you look at your surroundings and you see them clearly, thanks to the ocular stabilising function of the VOR. But what would happen if you decided to check the time on your wristwatch as you walked? The VOR would effectively take your eyes away from your watch as you turned. A mechanism exists that is capable of suppressing the VOR *when you want your eyes to focus on an object that rotates with you*, in this case your watch (Figure 1.8).

All the available evidence, from physiological and clinical studies, indicates that VOR-suppression and smooth-pursuit mechanisms are very similar if not identical. This is easy to visualise if you think of the different ways to follow a moving object, say a tennis ball. You can follow the ball with your eyes alone ('smooth pursuit') or you can follow it moving your eyes and head – in this latter case you have to suppress your VOR in order to be able to keep your eyes on the ball.

The practical importance of understanding the similarity of processes underlying smooth pursuit and VOR suppression lies in the fact that lesions that affect one system affect the other similarly. Since pursuit and VOR suppression by definition involve vision, visual attention, target selection and voluntary fixation, it goes almost without saying that such lesions are only and always central (i.e. in the brain). The message is that peripheral vestibular disorders spare VOR suppression and pursuit, whereas central disorders usually involve pursuit and VOR suppression. (For examination see Figure 2.5.)

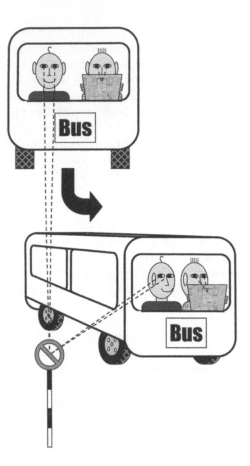

Figure 1.8 Vestibulo-ocular reflex (VOR) and VOR suppression. The person looking at the road sign while the bus turns round stabilises his eyes on the target with the VOR. The other person keeps his eyes on the newspaper by way of suppressing his VOR.

Smooth pursuit

This system allows the following of an object that moves in the visual field. If the moving object covers a large area of the visual field it can be called an optokinetic stimulus. In humans, both pursuit and optokinetic mechanisms are mediated largely by the cerebral cortex and the cerebellum and, therefore, the distinction between the two is not of practical importance. In animals, particularly those with poorly developed foveas and no smooth-pursuit system, optokinetic is a brainstem-based system capable of aiding the VOR. The anatomical bases of pursuit, optokinetic and VOR suppression in humans are similar, and abnormalities in these systems have identical significance.

As noted earlier these systems have a low-frequency response; that is, they work optimally at low frequencies (< 0.5 Hz) and low velocities (< 50 deg/s). At low target velocity, say 10 deg/s, eye velocity matches target velocity perfectly well, and this is sometimes defined as 'unity gain' (gain being defined as the ratio between eye velocity and target velocity). As the target velocity increases the eye velocity cannot keep up, so a small saccade is produced to catch up with the target. This is a normal process but, when smooth-pursuit pathways are affected, much of the visual tracking is done with saccades rather than with slow-phase pursuit. The clinical appearance of pursuit is therefore not 'smooth' at all but jerky, 'cogwheel' or 'broken'.

Saccades and quick phases of nystagmus

Saccades are fast refixation eye movements, with velocities of up to 500 deg/s. Their velocity is directly proportional to the size of the saccade but velocity is not under voluntary control. There are different types of saccades. Some of them are 'automatic' or reflexive, for instance in response to an unexpected sound or visual target; some of them are voluntary, such as saccades in the dark or in response to voluntary commands ('right', 'left', etc.) as investigated in the clinic.

The pathways mediating saccades are also widespread, as for pursuit movements. The high-frequency burst of neural activity required to accelerate the eye to the high velocities that saccades have is generated in the reticular formation of the brainstem. There are two main reticular centres, a pontine saccade generator responsible for horizontal saccades, and a midbrain one for vertical saccades. Lesions to either of these produce slow saccades and quick phases of nystagmus in the appropriate plane.

Multisensory integration

Summary

- Vestibular compensation is an adaptive process whereby symptoms and signs of an acute peripheral vestibular lesion gradually disappear. It depends on visual, proprioceptive and remaining vestibular inputs as well as on CNS plasticity.
- There is considerable overlap between the processes of spatial orientation and postural control. Proprioceptive, visual and vestibular mechanisms operate at both cortical (perceptual) and spinal (motor) levels.
- Sensory reweighting allows adequate balance control when one sensory input is unavailable or unreliable.

Many sensory inputs contribute to spatial orientation and balance control, in particular proprioceptive, vestibular and visual. Individual stimulation of each of these systems is capable of generating eye movements and postural responses. However, in normal circumstances these three sensory inputs are activated simultaneously, rather than individually, and this converging information interacts at virtually all levels in the neural axis.

Sensory conflict

Figure 1.9 shows that even in the simple case of a person turning his or her head sideways there is convergent input from the semicircular canals, the cervico-proprioceptive system and the visual system. Usually, the information conveyed is congruent, as in the case shown in the figure, where each sensory channel is indicating a head turn. It is believed that the sense of discomfort, malaise and nausea observed both during motion sickness and vestibular disorders arises, at least partly, due to the presence of what is called 'sensory conflict'.

Sensory conflict arises in various normal circumstances but usually for brief periods of time – for instance, conditions in which the VOR is suppressed as discussed above. A specific example is reading on a bus. Here, your vestibular system tells your brain that you are moving but your visual input, which in this example is self-referenced as you read, tells your brain that you are not (Figure 1.8).

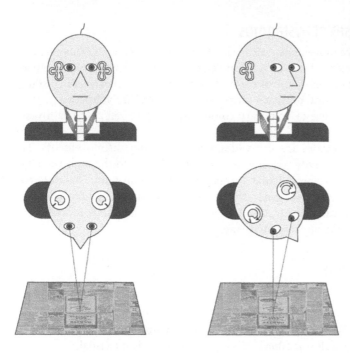

Figure 1.9 Multisensory integration. A person turning his head while reading a newspaper stimulates the vestibular system, the neck muscular and proprioceptive systems and the visual system. In this figure all inputs are congruent. In the example shown in Figure 1.8, however, the person reading the newspaper experiences 'sensory conflict' since the vestibular system signals head rotation but the visual system does not.

It is not clear why sensory conflict during motion should lead to nausea and vomiting. It has been argued that it may be a warning signal indicating that the circumstances in which you find yourself are not right and that you should, perhaps literally, abandon ship.

Vestibular disease, such as acute unilateral lesions, also creates sensory conflict. To start with there is vertigo, a continuous sensation of rotation that is not corroborated by any other sensory input. This may be the reason why some patients prefer to close their eyes. There is also a conflict between expected effects of movement and what is actually perceived. For instance, normally a head turn will be signalled by both labyrinths but, in unilateral disease, one input is suddenly absent. This may be one of the reasons why patients prefer to keep their head still.

However, sensorimotor conflict alone does not explain many aspects of the patients' symptoms. For instance, overstimulation of the CNS by congruent visuo-vestibular motion input also produces motion sickness as one would get on a ship if out on the deck and looking at the horizon. Probably an overstimulation mechanism also operates in spontaneous vestibular vertigo. This may explain why brief attacks of vertigo, as in BPPV, rarely lead to vomiting but vomiting is common in longer-duration vertigo attacks such as in vestibular neuritis or Ménière's disease.

Vestibular compensation

An acute unilateral vestibular lesion produces distressing vertigo, nystagmus, nausea and loss of postural balance. Even when the lesion is permanent and total, symptoms begin to improve in a few days and, in a few weeks, patients feel near normal. The nystagmus and tendency to fall to one side recovers and the intolerance to head movements gradually recovers in most patients. Since this recovery is not mediated by regrowth of the damaged inner ear the process is described as central vestibular compensation. This process, one of the best examples of central adaptation and plasticity by the CNS, depends on the remaining intact sensory inputs (contralateral vestibular, visual and proprioceptive) and a number of central integrating structures, including the vestibular nuclei and the cerebellum. Little is known on how higher-order mechanisms, such as the cortex, participate in this process.

From a clinical perspective it is most important to be aware that vestibular compensation is an active adaptive process and that rehabilitation works because it promotes vestibular compensation. Additional sensory problems (polyneuropathy, visual defects) or central problems (age, cerebrovascular disease) and excessive physical rest conspire against full recovery of a peripheral vestibular disorder and thus contribute to long-term dizzy symptoms.

Spatial orientation and postural control

Spatial orientation and postural control share many features despite the former being a perceptual process and the latter a motor process. The two are based, essentially, on the same sensory inputs – vestibular, visual and somatosensory – and central integration thereof. At the extreme, one can stand up only if one knows which way is up!

This next example illustrates the multisensory interaction present in postural and orientation control. Imagine yourself standing on a car facing the direction of the upcoming motion. As the car accelerates forward, your eyes see the world moving backwards; your otolith system senses the linear acceleration and your proprioceptive system is stimulated accordingly (e.g. your body will tend to fall backwards, creating a stretch stimulus of the anterior muscles of the leg). Each of these sensory inputs will activate parallel processes in the CNS: cortical mechanisms for spatial orientation and lower-level mechanisms generating reflexes and complex motor responses that enable you to stay upright as the car accelerates. It is easy to imagine, then, that stimulation of each sensory channel can produce disorientation and postural imbalance, and this has been demonstrated empirically. For instance, tendon vibration or visual motion stimuli create a sense of movement, spatial disorientation and unsteadiness.

Sensory reweighting

An important feature of the orientation–postural systems is the phenomenon of sensory weighting, that is, how much importance or 'weight' is attached to each sensory input at any one time. The simplest example is orienting or balancing with eyes open or closed. Clearly one puts a lot of weight on vision in the eyes-open and none in the eyes-closed condition. In disease, a relevant example for this book is that of a patient with a vestibular lesion. In vestibular patients, as the process of vestibular compensation sets in, there is an increase in the weight given to visual and proprioceptive inputs. Whilst this mechanism undoubtedly aids vestibular recovery, excessive reliance on visual input (or 'visual dependence') makes patients prone to disorientation and imbalance in situations where visual input is conflicting or unreliable, for instance a moving visual surround (see page 134).

The sensory reweighting process works optimally when the three main sensory inputs are working normally. If only two inputs are available, then *sensory weighting is suboptimal.*

A patient with no proprioception can stay upright with eyes open but falls over on eye closure (the basis of the Romberg test). Patients with bilateral or severe unilateral vestibular disorders can walk quite well, with eyes open and full proprioceptive input; if there is an additional polyneuropathy, or if they stand on foam with eyes closed as a clinical test, they fall over. Remember that in old age all three sensory inputs, as well as central integrative structures, are degraded; so it is easy to see why balance problems are so common in the elderly.

Chapter 2

Symptoms and examination of the patient with vertigo and dizziness

History-taking is, without a doubt, the most important component in the diagnostic puzzle of the dizzy patient and may lead to correct classification in two-thirds of patients. Most of the remaining third become clear after thorough clinical examination. Technical investigations can add supportive evidence but are rarely diagnostic. Tables 2.1, 2.2 and 2.3 provide an overview of how symptoms, clinical findings and testing procedures can be used for the diagnostic process.

Table 2.1 Symptoms as a clue to diagnosis

Feature	Suspected diagnosis
Presentation type of dizziness	
Rotational vertigo	Acute vestibular disorder (central or peripheral)
Positional vertigo	Benign paroxysmal positional vertigo (BPPV), migraine, central positional vertigo
Unsteadiness	Bilateral vestibular dysfunction, neurological disorder (e.g. polyneuropathy, myelopathy, normal-pressure hydrocephalus, cerebral small-vessel disease, cerebellar disorder)
Non-specific dizziness	Orthostatic hypotension, drug toxicity, psychogenic
Duration of attacks	
Seconds	Vestibular paroxysms, cardiac arrhythmia, BPPV
Few minutes	TIAs, panic attacks, migraine
20 minutes to several hours	Ménière attacks, migraine
Days to weeks	Vestibular neuritis, brainstem/cerebellar stroke or demyelination, migraine
Persistent	Fixed neurological deficit, bilateral vestibular failure, chronic intoxication, psychogenic
Triggers	
Changes of head position	BPPV, other positional vertigo
Menstruation, sleep deprivation	Migraine
Moving visual patterns	Visual vertigo (visually induced dizziness)
Elevators and other close spaces, crowds, heights, leaving the house	Panic attacks
Loud noises, Valsalva manoeuvres	Fistula syndromes

Table 2.1 (*cont.*)

Feature	Suspected diagnosis
Standing up	Orthostatic hypotension
Associated symptoms	
Photophobia, headache or visual auras	Migraine
Hearing loss, tinnitus, fullness in the ear	Ménière's disease, autoimmune inner-ear disease, acoustic neuroma
Blackening out of vision, syncope	Vasovagal reaction, orthostatic hypotension, cardiac arrhythmia
Red eyes, skin rashes, renal disease, arthritis	Autoimmune inner-ear disease
Palpitations, choking, trembling, catastrophic thoughts, panic	Anxiety disorder
Diplopia, dysarthria, numbness, paresis, clouded consciousness	Posterior fossa lesion (including ischemia), basilar migraine

TIA = transient ischaemic attack

Table 2.2 Examination of the dizzy patient

Examination	Interpretation
Spontaneous nystagmus	Peripheral or central vestibular disorder Peripheral: horizontal–torsional, increases without fixation Central: any direction (up, down, torsional, horizontal)
Clinical VOR assessment (head-thrust or head-impulse test)	Detects major peripheral vestibular loss (i.e. > 60%)
Eye movements (pursuit, saccades, VOR suppression)	Abnormalites indicate central lesion
Positional manoeuvre	Identifies benign paroxysmal positional vertigo (and only rarely posterior fossa lesion)
Romberg test: normal unidirectional fall variable swaying with eyes open swaying after eye closure	 In most dizzy patients Acute vestibular lesion Cerebellar/brainstem lesion Dorsal-column spinal disorder/large-fibre neuropathy
Gait abnormalities	Cerebellar, parkinsonian, spastic, apraxic, neuropathic disorders
Gait with eyes closed or Unterberger test	Ipsilesional deviation in peripheral lesions
Postural responses to trunk pushes	Impaired in parkinsonian syndromes and small-vessel white-matter disease.

VOR = vestibulo-ocular reflex

Table 2.3 Laboratory investigations for dizzy patients

Test	Interpretation
Pure-tone audiometry	Essential for Ménière's disease (often low-frequency loss) Red flag for acoustic neuroma Normal in most other vestibular disorders
Brainstem auditory-evoked responses (BAER)	Useful screening for acoustic neuroma in patients with unilateral auditory symptoms
Caloric and rotational tests (including vHIT)	Caloric canal paresis or unilateral vHIT abnormality: lack of response from one ear, often observed in peripheral vestibular disorders Directional preponderance (on caloric or rotational tests): indicates vestibular asymmetry – non-specific
Eye-movement recordings (electro-/video-oculography)	Do not replace clinical eye-movement examination! May help to detect central dysfunction
MRI consider when: central symptoms/signs atypical positional nystagmus progressive unilateral sensorineural hearing loss	Identification of posterior fossa lesion (MRI superior to CT)

MRI = magnetic resonance imaging; CT = computed tomography; vHIT = video Head Impulse Test

Symptoms

Most diseases causing dizziness have distinct symptoms, or combinations of symptoms. This applies to conditions such as benign paroxysmal positional vertigo (BPPV), vestibular neuritis, vestibular migraine, Ménière's disease, vertebrobasilar transient ischaemic attacks (TIAs) or syncopal episodes. Details of the symptoms of these disorders can be found in the specific sections of this book. Here we will give a description of the components that are common to some frequently seen disorders and some practical help to differentiate them.

Vertigo

Vertigo is an illusion of movement. The common variety, rotational or 'true' vertigo, indicates disease of the semicircular canals or their central nervous system (CNS) connections. Patients with vertigo say that they, or the room, spin around. When patients actually see the world spinning around it is very likely that they have nystagmus during the vertigo. Although some clinicians give less value to patients' reports of 'something spinning inside the head', we have seen many patients with genuine vestibular disease (e.g. BPPV) describing their vertigo in such a way. Patients with 'true' vertigo usually have accompanying symptoms such as imbalance, unsteadiness (or veering) of gait, nausea and vomiting.

Dizziness, or related terms such as giddiness, are difficult to define precisely for both patients and doctors. Other descriptions provided by patients are light-headedness, feeling off-balance, rocking sensations, and 'walking on cotton wool'. These can indicate disease of the vestibular system, particularly in non-acute stages; but general medical disease (e.g. anaemia, hypoglycaemia, cardiac) or psychogenic disorders are also likely. It is useful to ask the patient to try to compare the symptom to anything that he or she may have experienced in everyday life. Then patients often describe 'true' vertigo or vestibular-mediated sensations, such as being drunk, or on a merry-go-round or a boat in rough seas, or car-sickness. Often, vague dizziness is a transitional state, between an acute vestibular episode and full recovery.

For diagnostic purposes it is vital to identify the presentation type, duration, triggers and associated symptoms in all patients with dizziness or vertigo (Table 2.1). Note that all names of specific disorders mentioned below can be found in the index and then traced to sections describing them in detail.

Presentation type

As soon as you see a patient with dizziness try to establish whether the problem is (a) a single, acute episode of vertigo, (b) recurrent or episodic vertigo dizziness, or (c) chronic sensations of unsteadiness or dizziness. The most frequent cause of a single vertigo attack is vestibular neuritis but you should always consider stroke as a possibility. Other causes are traumatic or infectious. The most frequent cause of recurrent spontaneous vertigo is migraine; others include Ménière's disease, vestibular paroxysms, vertebrobasilar TIAs and episodic ataxias. Positional vertigo is typically caused by BPPV but occasionally by migraine and rarely by a posterior fossa lesion. Unsteadiness may result from bilateral vestibular loss but is more commonly related to neurological disorders such as cerebellar disease, parkinsonism, myelopathy, neuropathy or cerebral small-vessel disease. Non-specific dizziness can be caused by general medical disorders, chronic drug toxicity, minor vestibular dysfunction or psychological factors.

Duration

Vertigo duration is typically seconds in BPPV, hours in migraine and Ménière's disease, days in vestibular neuritis. It is important to determine the duration of the actual rotational sensation ('the bad spinning') since patients tend to include the aftermath (malaise, nausea) in the total duration. This explains why so many patients with typical BPPV are adamant that their attacks last up to half an hour.

Triggers

Of all possible triggers, head positioning is the most useful, but certain head positions are much more revealing than others. Consider these two statements: (1) the only way to achieve a new position of the head is by moving it, and (2) the vestibular apparatus is the system specialised to detect head movements. Hence, it is hardly surprising that *any* change in position of the head will make *any* vestibular disorder symptomatic. From this we can conclude two useful things. First, dizziness worsening on head movements is likely to be of vestibular origin. Second, more importantly, positional vertigo is not just getting dizzy on head movements.

The specific situations that are useful for the diagnosis of positional vertigo, particularly BPPV, involve reorientation of the head with respect to the *gravity vector*. There are many such situations, for instance standing up from the lying-down position. However, the trigger situations most useful for diagnosing BPPV are lying down or turning over in bed. This is so because orthostatic hypotension can provoke dizziness on standing up but not on lying or turning over in bed. Reciprocally, a patient being dizzy on standing up from the sitting-down position is more likely to have orthostatic hypotension than positional vertigo, since the head is not reoriented with respect to gravity from sitting to standing (Figure 2.1).

A common, related, misconception is that patients who report dizziness on moving the head suffer from vague disorders such as 'vertebrobasilar insufficiency' or 'cervical vertigo'. The issue will be discussed in Chapter 5, but at this stage just consider our two earlier statements: the only way to achieve a new position of the head is by moving it, and the vestibular apparatus is a head-movement detection system. Now add a third statement: (3) most head movements are accomplished by neck movements and it follows that *most vestibular disorders will become symptomatic on neck movements*. In fact, most patients referred to us with provisional diagnoses of 'vertebrobasilar insufficiency' or 'cervical vertigo' suffer from vestibular disorders, including BPPV.

Other vertigo triggers are very specific but rare, because the underlying diseases are uncommon. Loud sounds and Valsalva manoeuvres can trigger vestibular symptoms,

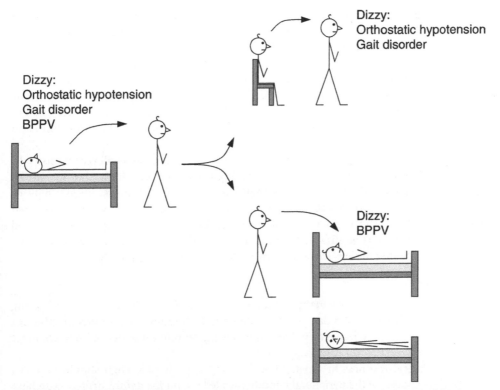

Figure 2.1 Dizziness after getting up can imply orthostatic hypotension, a gait disorder or BPPV. If the dizziness is provoked by standing up from sitting (top right), orthostatic hypotension or a gait disorder is more likely than BPPV because head orientation remains unchanged with respect to gravity in this situation. In contrast, dizziness after lying down or turning over in bed (bottom right) usually indicates BPPV.

including lateropulsion and oscillopsia, in the superior canal dehiscence syndrome. A labyrinthine fistula, with acute vertigo and unilateral deafness, can be secondary to head trauma or strong Valsalva effort (e.g. heavy object lifting or cough attack). Alcohol or exercise can trigger vertigo in patients with episodic or paroxysmal ataxias.

Other triggers are encountered frequently but are not so specific. In some patients with chronic dizziness, environments with repetitive visual patterns or visual motion can aggravate or trigger dizziness (visually induced dizziness or 'visual vertigo'). In patients with psychogenic conditions, certain social situations or specific triggers (lifts, small rooms, aeroplanes) can trigger panic symptoms including dizziness.

Associated symptoms

Unsteadiness

During any episode of rotational vertigo the patient is also unsteady. During acute and intense episodes there is an irresistible tendency to fall in one direction; examples are a BPPV episode whilst standing up ('hanging clothes on the washing line'), the first day in vestibular neuritis, Ménière's attacks, and lateral medullary (Wallenberg) syndrome. Usually, this body lateropulsion is towards the hypoactive vestibular apparatus or nucleus; but remember that BPPV and the initial phase of a Ménière's attack represent vestibular hyperactivity, not hypoactivity.

A sense of unsteadiness may persist in the chronic phase in most peripheral unilateral vestibular disorders. On specific questioning, however, most patients will acknowledge that this is only a subjective sensation and that friends, relatives or colleagues have never noticed anything wrong.

Patients with bilateral vestibular disorders, when vestibular loss is total or subtotal (see page 141), report gait unsteadiness particularly when walking on irregular ground or in the dark. (NB: bilateral vestibular failure can be insidious and idiopathic, so always enquire about darkness in a patient with an unexplained gait unsteadiness, and about oscillopsia on walking.)

Patients with a variety of non-vestibular neurological gait disorders will report unsteadiness, sometimes leading to falls after trivial tripping over. The neurologist, but not necessarily ENT specialists, will be familiar with these disorders and with the additional signs or symptoms leading to correct diagnosis. Except in cerebellar disease, where disordered cerebellar–vestibular interaction might provoke vestibular symptoms, most patients will acknowledge that there is no dizziness 'in the head' and that the trouble is 'in the legs'. So, specifically ask whether the legs feel weak, heavy, clumsy or numb, or have 'pins and needles'.

Aural symptoms

It must be borne in mind that many common causes of vertigo do not produce hearing symptoms (e.g. BPPV, vestibular neuritis, migraine). Auditory symptoms helpful for diagnosis are not actually frequent in the clinic. Owing to referral patterns, they are more conspicuous in ENT than in neurology clinics.

Acute unilateral deafness in a patient with a first episode of vertigo should be taken seriously. Severe cases of the peripheral condition called *idiopathic sudden deafness* can have vertigo. The same applies for viral labyrinthitis of known (e.g. mumps) or unknown aetiology. If the symptoms develop after physical effort a fistula is almost certain, and rest, observation and a possible exploration are indicated. These conditions are emergencies with respect to the outcome of the hearing loss. In contrast, a posterior-circulation vascular episode, typically the anterior inferior cerebellar artery syndrome, has all the potential life-threatening implications of any stroke. These vascular episodes add pathognomonic brain-stem symptoms (diplopia, ataxia, numbness) but these should be actively elicited as patients can be overwhelmed by the vertigo and deafness.

Fluctuating aural pressure, tinnitus and hearing loss are reported by patients with Ménière's disease. However, it must be stressed that in an unselected clinical environment Ménière's disease is rare. In the context of repetitive vertebrobasilar TIA episodes, patients may have tinnitus or hearing loss together with other brainstem symptoms. The presence of phono- (and photo-) phobia is useful for the diagnosis of migraine-related vertigo. Although acoustic neuromas and other tumours usually do not cause vertigo or unsteadiness, the presence of unilateral progressive tinnitus and deafness should raise a red flag.

Trivial and age-related aural symptoms are very common in the general population. When patients report that 'My wife/husband says that I have the TV too loud' or 'Yes, when I am quietly in bed I can hear a hissing sound in my ears', audiological investigations are usually unrevealing (but reassuring nevertheless). The label of Ménière's disease is so often stuck to the patient with vertigo and trivial hearing symptoms that the clinician should refrain from suggesting this diagnosis to the patient until further investigations are completed. We spend more time saying, 'No, you don't have Ménière's disease', than saying, 'What you have is called Ménière's disease'.

Less frequent symptoms
Disequilibrium

Patients with balance disorders can be unsteady objectively ('they look unsteady') and subjectively ('they feel unsteady'). Patients who feel and look unsteady but have no head sensations such as dizziness, vertigo or 'about to faint' presyncopal feelings are also seen in the clinic. This is often called disequilibrium. When presented with the question 'Is the problem in the head or the legs?' patients with disequilibrium tend to acknowledge the latter. They will also report no balance symptoms when seated. These patients may have a neurological disorder of gait including weakness, spasticity, numbness, slowness, shakiness or incoordination of the legs due to lesions almost anywhere in the peripheral or central nervous system; some examples are polyneuropathy, spinal cord, brainstem, cerebellar or hemispheric lesion, hydrocephalus, or parkinsonian or other movement disorders. Patients may have falls; these are more common in patients with disequilibrium due to a neurological gait disorder than in vestibular patients. The neurological and neuro-otological examination (in particular eye movements and gait) will usually identify the non-peripheral vestibular origin of the problem. This is seen in Chapter 7 but, in essence, if a patient has normal gait (including gait with eyes open, closed and tandem heel-to-toe) and normal eye movements it is unlikely that his or her unsteadiness is due to a neurological problem. Falls due to loss of consciousness and drop attacks are also discussed in Chapter 7.

Oscillopsia

Oscillopsia is the illusion that the visual world is moving or oscillating. It must be mentioned that the specific illusion that the visual environment is rotating is usually called vertigo (or 'objective vertigo' as opposed to the illusion of self-rotation or 'subjective' vertigo). (NB: in German-speaking countries objective vertigo may be called oscillopsia.)

Patients with severe bilateral loss of vestibular function (e.g. post-meningitis or by gentamicin ototoxicity) report oscillopsia when they move, walk, run or ride in a car. This is due to the lack of image stabilisation during head movements, the specific function of the vestibulo-ocular reflex (VOR). Patients with a variety of nystagmus also report oscillopsia but not necessarily related to their own motion. Essentially, oscillopsia develops when the retinal image is not stable, because the eyes move either too much (e.g. nystagmus) or not enough (loss of VOR).

It is useful to enquire directly about the presence of oscillopsia, particularly in patients describing visual shimmering, blurring or odd visual symptoms. One can quickly enquire about diplopia and oscillopsia routinely by asking patients if they have double or wobbly vision. Having established the presence of oscillopsia, the critical question for diagnosis is *when* the oscillopsia occurs (Table 2.4). If it is related to patient movement, the cause is almost certainly the loss of the vestibulo-ocular reflex (see page 141, video clip 02.01). If it develops after adopting a particular head position, the cause is likely to be a positional nystagmus (see page 108, video clip 02.20); we had a patient with a position-sensitive upbeat nystagmus who could not read whilst supine as all the lines would jumble up. If the oscillopsia is always there, it may be due to an acquired neurological nystagmus (e.g. downbeat nystagmus, video clip 07.02) or ocular oscillation (e.g. opsoclonus). If the oscillopsia is paroxysmal – usually intense but lasting for a few seconds only – the patient can have a vestibular paroxysm, a paroxysmal nystagmus (usually secondary to a brainstem vascular lesion) or the condition called *voluntary nystagmus*, which is essentially a psychological conversion disorder characterised by fast paroxysmal horizontal ocular oscillations.

Table 2.4 Oscillopsia: diagnostic algorithm

During movements of the head	Absent VOR: bilateral loss of vestibular function (e.g. ototoxic, post-meningitic, idiopathic)
Triggered by movements of the head	Central positional nystagmus: brainstem–cerebellar disease (e.g. positional downbeat nystagmus)
At rest (not significantly associated to movement) Paroxysmal	Sound-induced: Tullio phenomenon (superior canal dehiscence) Vestibular paroxysms: vestibular paroxysmia, Vestibular nuclear lesions Ocular flutter Microflutter Voluntary nystagmus Monocular: superior oblique myokymia
Continuous	Nystagmus due to brainstem or cerebellar lesion (e.g. acquired pendular nystagmus, upbeat, downbeat, torsional) Pseudonystagmus (head tremor + absent VOR)

VOR = vestibulo-ocular reflex

Video 02.01 – Oscillopsia due to bilateral vestibular failure
This video clip was taken by holding the video camera and jogging on the spot. This is an attempt to simulate how a patient with absent vestibulo-ocular reflex (VOR) sees the world when walking energetically, running or travelling on a vehicle on a bumpy road. As simulated in the video clip the oscillopsia in patients with absent VOR is only present when the patient is moving and it stops when the subject remains stationary.

Brainstem symptoms

The presence of brainstem and cerebellar symptoms is the rule in patients with vertigo or imbalance due to vertebrobasilar strokes, TIAs, multiple sclerosis or posterior fossa tumours. They include double vision, speech problems, limb or gait ataxia, swallowing difficulty and facial numbness or weakness. The time course and presentation is directly related to the underlying disease: episodic in TIAs, relapsing–remitting in multiple sclerosis, progressive in tumours and acute in strokes. Although the additional symptoms and signs in these conditions make confusion with a vestibular disorder unlikely, acute small lesions in the intra-axial portion of the eighth nerve, vestibular nuclei or cerebellum can mimic the picture of a vestibular neuritis. In vestibular neuritis, nystagmus and lateropulsion are expected. If in addition the eye-movement examination (see later) is not quite normal, or if in doubt for any other reason (facial numbness, atrial fibrillation), imaging procedures are warranted.

Detailed interrogation and examination of the patient with brainstem lesions is rich and useful for establishing lesion site, diagnosis, prognosis and follow-up. However, it will not be dealt with in detail here as our remit is the diagnosis and management of dizziness and vertigo.

Loss of consciousness

Loss of consciousness is rare amongst dizzy patients, except when the cause is haemodynamic. Thus, patients with syncope due to heart arrhythmia, vasovagal symptoms or autonomic nervous system disorders with orthostatic hypotension do report dizziness or vertigo before they pass out. It is therefore important to enquire about previous heart history, palpitations or tightness in the chest which would point to a heart disorder. Needless to say, in the presence of these symptoms priority should be given to cardiological rather than neuro-otological investigations. However, always bear in mind that heart and vestibular disorders are very common and many patients have both.

Sweating, hot or cold bodily sensations, clammy hands, bilateral tinnitus and 'greying out' of vision are reported by patients with hypotensive episodes as in vasovagal syncope and orthostatic hypotension. Witnesses can report that patients look pale or off colour during the faints. Typically, patients regain consciousness within seconds of falling or lying down as brain irrigation is restored. With repeated episodes many patients learn to recognise the trigger situations and prevent the episodes by lying down or sitting with the head lowered between the legs. Such situations can include hot and stuffy rooms, cognitive triggers (e.g. sight of blood), trivial pain, or standing upright quickly or for long periods of time. Many patients only report dizziness, and the accompanying symptoms described above, but do not faint in these situations. These presyncopal syndromes are difficult to diagnose, even with formal autonomic function tests. The clinician should therefore enquire actively about trigger situations, previous history of fainting episodes, and whether lying down has any (beneficial) effect.

Patients with hypoglycaemia – due to medication in diabetic patients or more rarely insulin-secreting tumours – can be dizzy and pass out. Most diabetic patients recognise this and can prevent the loss of consciousness with appropriate foods. Most patients with actual loss of consciousness would have been taken to a hospital emergency service and their blood glucose measured, but if in doubt, measure it again.

Vestibular epilepsy is not a well-defined entity. Since the work of Penfield with direct electrical stimulation of the cortex in awake patients, we know that rotational vertigo can be elicited by activation of the temporal lobe. We also know that isolated cases of acute vascular lesions of the temporal cortex producing vertigo have been reported, and that patients with epilepsy can include brief vertigo in their aura. However, recurrent vertigo, without other epileptic phenomena, is not likely to be due to epilepsy. The term *vestibular paroxysm* or *paroxysmia* (see Chapter 4) implies brief episodes of vertigo and/or oscillopsia due to irritation of the vestibular nerve or nuclei in the brainstem, and these patients do not lose consciousness.

Finally, some patients occasionally report that, during the intense vertigo in the acute phase of a vestibular neuritis or Ménière's disease, they 'think' they passed out. It is very difficult to know exactly what happens in these circumstances, but one suspects that the combination of a new terrifying symptom, perhaps aggravated by panic or dehydration if vomiting has occurred, or syncope in the patient with a propensity, may be at play. When witnesses are available, they usually describe that communication with the patient was precarious but possible, indicating that no complete loss of consciousness was present.

Essentials of the clinical examination

Since many different specialists as well as generalists see patients with dizziness, it is inevitable that the emphasis of the examination will be different from doctor to doctor. Some specialists will be consulted to make sure that there is no ear, brain or heart cause for a patient's symptoms. Fair enough. The doctor in charge of the patient, however, should be aware that this approach is a non-winning formula *because standard ENT, neurological or cardiological investigations are often negative in dizzy patients*. The general physician, geriatrician, audiological physician, neurologist or ENT surgeon who wants to stay in overall control of the patient has to be prepared to cross over specialties.

It is easy to pontificate that all patients with dizziness need a full cardiological, neuro-logical and ENT examination, but the hit rate would be very small. A more realistic approach, restating the obvious, is to say that patients with organ-specific symptoms should have that organ examined. Patients with dizziness related to chest pain, palpitations, faintness or orthostatic positioning must have a cardiovascular examination, and blood pressure and pulse measurements supine and immediately on standing up, and repeatedly while standing up for three minutes. Patients with aural pressure, fullness, pain or discharge and/or tinnitus and hearing loss should have the ears examined with an auriscope (otoscope). Patients with brainstem symptoms (see above) or weakness, slowness, clumsiness or numbness in the limbs need to have a neurological examination. If in doubt, or when there are clear findings on examination, an appropriate specialist opinion is warranted. The same applies to general medical conditions capable of producing dizziness; but here, routine blood tests including glycaemia, ESR, blood counts, liver function and lipids are a useful screening tool.

Provided there are no clear organ-specific indicators in the history, and often there are none, the usual question is whether the problem is a central (CNS) or peripheral (labyrin-thine) vestibular disorder. (NB: the eighth nerve may be considered 'central' by ENT specialists and 'peripheral' by neurologists.) Some preliminary rules of thumb can be given here. A patient without brainstem symptoms and normal eye movements is very unlikely to have a central disorder. A patient with clear brainstem or limb symptoms has a central disorder until proven otherwise. A patient with abnormal eye movements, even if the history 'sounds' peripheral, is likely to have a central disorder. (NB: we mean clinically observable abnormal eye movements other than a peripheral vestibular nystagmus, and *not* obscure electronystagmographic findings.) It follows that a vital part of the diagnosis relies on the eye-movement examination and that it is equally important to establish whether the movements are abnormal or normal.

Eye-movement examination

Even if you have access to vestibular testing facilities, these do not replace the clinical examination of eye movements. Once you acquire a routine it should not take more than three to four minutes to complete. Movements of the eyes belong to very specific subsystems and these need to be examined separately. The examination should consist of a search for spontaneous and gaze-evoked nystagmus, convergence, pursuit, saccadic and vestibular eye movements (video clips 02.02–02.27). Positional nystagmus is such an essential part of the investigation of the dizzy patient that it will be presented separately here and again in Chapter 5.

Nystagmus: the starting point of the investigation

Primary gaze ('spontaneous nystagmus')

The patient is asked to fixate on a stationary object presented straight ahead. The object has to be clearly visible, i.e. it must not be tiny or be too close to the eyes in a presbyopic individual. Ask the patient if he/she can see the object (finger, pen) clearly, particularly if glasses have been removed. Look for nystagmus actively and help to keep one of the patient's eyes wider with your finger and/or thumb. (The way to help patients keep their eyes open is shown in Figure 5.1 during a positional manoeuvre and in many video clips in this chapter.) If there is nystagmus, note the *type of oscillation*: intercalated fast and slow phases, or jerk nystagmus; slow-phase-alone sinusoidal oscillation of the eyes, or pendular nystagmus; or fast-phase-alone oscillation, or saccadic oscillations. Also note the *plane of the oscillation*: horizontal, vertical, torsional ('rotatory') or combinations thereof.

Gaze-evoked nystagmus

Take the fixation target some 30 degrees to the right, left, up and down of primary gaze (30 degrees is approximately three hand widths, or 12 fingers across, at an average fixation distance of 30 cm) (video clips 02.02 and 02.03). If you go too far, apart from the fact that the patient's nose will obstruct vision in the adducting eye, many normal people will have nystagmus. Stay a few seconds in each position; if you are in doubt stay as long as you need.

Video 02.02 – Clinical examination: convergence and search for spontaneous and gaze-evoked nystagmus
For convergence examination the target is brought closer to the subject's eyes. For spontaneous nystagmus the eyes are observed in the primary position. For detection of gaze-evoked nystagmus the fixation target is moved to the right, left, up and down. A deviation of approximately 30° as shown, is advisable. The eyes can be manually opened for optimal visibility.

Video 02.03 – Examination for convergence and search for spontaneous and gaze-evoked nystagmus
Note the good convergence of the eyes on to the near target and the absence of spontaneous nystagmus or ocular oscillations in primary gaze. Furthermore, there is no gaze-evoked nystagmus on ± 30° deviation to the right, left, up or down.

Video 02.04 – Examination for gaze limitation
In contrast to examination of a spontaneous nystagmus, when investigating if there is a limitation of gaze in any direction the eye has to be taken as far out as possible.

Video 02.05 – Clinical examination of smooth pursuit
A clearly visible target presented at comfortable viewing distance for the subject is moved slowly and smoothly in the horizontal and vertical plane.

Video 02.06 – Normal smooth pursuit
Notice smooth tracking of the visual target by the normal subject.

Video 02.07 – Clinical examination of saccades
The subject is asked to look to the appearing finger and, in this case, given simultaneous verbal commands. Small saccades can be elicited by asking the subject to look between your index finger and thumb both horizontally and vertically. In this case the eye can be opened with the other hand of the examiner for optimal visibility of the patient's eyes.

Video 02.08 – Normal saccades
Note the fast, conjugate and accurate movements elicited in this case by simultaneous flicking of the examiner's fingers together with verbal commands.

Video 02.09 – Clinical examination of the vestibulo-ocular reflex (VOR) with the head-thrust manoeuvre
The patient, in this case a normal subject, fixates the examiner's nose while her head is abruptly rotated by the doctor's hands. The aim is to produce a brief, but fast head turn, while simultaneously being able to observe the patient's eyes carefully.

Video 02.10 – Normal head thrust (or head-impulse test)
Note how the subject's eyes under examination, remain fixed on the examiner's nose. Note that there are no 'catch-up' saccades. Examples of abnormal results during head-thrust tests in unilateral and bilateral patients with peripheral vestibular loss are given in video clips 02.13 – Abnormal head thrust to the right, and 02.14 – Bilaterally abnormal head-thrust test, respectively.

Video 02.11 – Doll's head-eye manoeuvre
This video clip shows a doll's head-eye manoeuvre during slow oscillation of the head in the horizontal and vertical plane. The subject fixates the examiner's nose.

Video 02.12 – Normal doll's head-eye manoeuvre
During the slow doll's head oscillation of the head, the eyes produce a slow and completely smooth movement compensating for the head movement induced by the examiner's hands.

Video 02.13 – Abnormal head-thrust test to the right
Patient with a near-total loss of vestibular function on the right (following a vestibular neuritis). Note the presence of corrective 'catch-up' saccades, indicative of an insufficient VOR, during head turns to the right. During left head turns the eyes remain stable on the fixation point (in this case the camera lens but, usually, the examiner's nose).

Video 02.14 – Bilaterally abnormal head-thrust test
Patient with bilateral complete loss of vestibular function. Note the presence of 'catch-up' saccades towards the fixation point during head thrusts to the right and left.

Video 02.15 – Normal VOR suppression
The subject is seated on an office swivel chair. The subject (in this case a normal subject) is oscillated while looking at his own thumbs. The close up images shows that the subject does not have nystagmus i.e. he manages to successfully suppress his own vestibular nystagmus. Still pictures of alternative ways of examining VOR suppression are shown in Figure 2.4 in the text.

Video 02.16 – Clinical examination: Hallpike to the left
The head is turned to the left and then the patient is brought back to the left-ear-down, head-hanging position. The head should remain at least 10–15 seconds in the head-down position because common forms of positional nystagmus have a latency. The eyes can always be helped to stay open manually by the examiner. Use your own nose as a target to the patient and place your nose in front of the eyes of the patient so that you can ensure that the eyes remain in primary gaze.

Video 02.17 – Clinical examination: Hallpike to the right
The head is turned to the right by 45° in the upright position and the patient is then quickly brought back to the right-ear-down, head-hanging position. Observe the subject's eyes for 15 seconds or so making sure that the patient's eyes remain in primary gaze but present your own nose as a target.

Video 02.18 – Clinical examination: sideways, or variant, Hallpike to the left
For an alternative way to do the left-ear-down positional manoeuvre, the patient (in this case a normal subject) is asked to turn the head some 45° to the right and then she is abruptly made to lay down sideways on her left. Notice that the final head position with this manoeuvre and the conventional left Hallpike are very similar (video clip 02.16 – Clinical examination: Hallpike to the left).

Video 02.19 – Clinical examination: sideways Hallpike to the right
The head is turned to the left and then the patient is quickly brought down sideways on to the right.

Video 02.20 – Positional downbeat nystagmus
The video clip shows two takes of a patient with positional downbeat nystagmus. First elicited during the straight-back positional manoeuvre. The second clip shows the same nystagmus during the conventional right-ear-down Hallpike manoeuvre.

Video 02.21 – Acquired pendular nystagmus
The video clip shows a patient with previous brainstem stroke (pontine) showing an irregular, mostly vertical pendular nystagmus.

Video 02.22 Gaze-evoked nysthagmus
The video clip shows a patient with cerebellar atrophy (SCA 6). Initially, in primary gaze there is no nystagmus. On gaze deviation to the right a gaze-evoked nystagmus appears. After returning to primary position a few small beats of left-beating nystagmus are seen. During deviation of the eyes to the left a slightly more prominent left-beating, gaze-evoked nystagmus is observed. Back in primary position, two or three small beats of right-beating nystagmus are observed. In this case the nystagmus evoked by lateral gaze is called gaze-evoked nystagmus and the nystagmus transiently seen after recentering gaze is called rebound nystagmus. More video clips of the same patient: 02.23 – Abnormal pursuit, and 02.24 – Abnormal VOR suppression.

Video 02.23 – Abnormal pursuit
Note that this patient's smooth pursuit is jerky when following the slowly moving target. The patient has cerebellar atrophy (SCA 6). Compare this to the normal subject in video clip 02.06 – Normal smooth pursuit. More video clips of the same patient: 02.22 – Gaze-evoked nystagmus and 02.24 – Abnormal VOR suppression.

Video 02.24 – Abnormal VOR suppression
The video clip shows a patient oscillating on a conventional swivel chair while attempting to fixate his own thumbs. Note that he does not succeed in keeping his eyes fully on his thumbs and he displays nystagmus during the oscillation. Compare this to the normal subject in video clip 02.15 – Normal VOR suppression. More video clips of the same patient: 02.22 – Gaze-evoked nystagmus and 02.23 – Abnormal pursuit.

Video 02.25 – Saccadic hypometria in Parkinson's disease
The video clip shows a patient with idiopathic Parkinson's disease fixating between the examiner's fingers on the patient's right and left. In the first half of the clip, the saccades are elicited by variable prompt and flicking of the examiner's fingers. In this situation the gaze performance is normal. However, the second half of the clip shows that on self-paced saccades, the saccades become markedly hypometric.

Video 02.26 – Saccadic hypermetria in cerebellar disease
The video shows a patient with cerebellar haematoma showing hypermetric saccades. Compare this to the normal subject in video clip 02.08 – Normal saccades.

Video 02.27 – Slow saccades
The video clip shows a patient with horizontal and vertical slow saccades, which is the main finding. (In addition, there is a small tendency for the left eye to diverge). Compare this to the normal subject in video clip 02.08 – Normal saccades.

Video 02.28 – Internuclear ophthalmoplegia (INO)
Examination of horizontal saccades in a patient with a diagnosis of multiple sclerosis. During saccades to the left one can observe that the right (adducting) eye is slower than the left (abducting) eye. At the end of the leftwards saccades the right eye does not fully adduct and gaze becomes disconjugate; note the left-eye nystagmus (abducting or 'ataxic' nystagmus) thus completing all features of a right INO. Saccades to the right are essentially normal, but a slight slowing of left-eye adduction can be detected, testimony to this patient's previous left INO.

Note the type and plane of eye oscillation. The amplitude of the oscillation is also important: some patients have a large-amplitude gaze-evoked nystagmus called *gaze paretic nystagmus* because they seem unable to keep the eyes on the target in the prescribed eccentric position (video clip 02.22). This usually results from ipsilateral brainstem or cerebellar lesions, and other CNS symptoms or signs often testify to this. In contrast, peripheral vestibular disorders produce a fine horizontal nystagmus; if large it is usually an enhancement of a nystagmus that is also observable in primary gaze (second-degree nystagmus).

We discuss the types and significance of nystagmus in the various clinical chapters of this book, according to the vertigo presentation (Chapters 3–7). Suffice it to say here that the only spontaneous nystagmus that can be accepted as of peripheral vestibular origin is horizontal (or horizontal with a minor torsional component) and unidirectional. In the acute stage of a vertigo attack the nystagmus can be present in primary gaze (second-degree), but as the patient improves it will be seen only with gaze deviation in the direction of the fast phase (first-degree) (see page 55 and video clip 03.01). This nystagmus could be central as well but, in this case, there will be other brainstem symptoms, signs or oculo-motor abnormalities. Any other nystagmus in an upright patient (i.e. different type and plane of oscillation) is central in origin. Table 2.5 gives an overview of common types of pathological nystagmus and their general clinical interpretation.

Convergence

The assessment of convergence is not particularly useful in the dizzy patient. It must be said, however, that nystagmus often increases in amplitude and is therefore more visible during the convergence effort (video clip 07.02). Therefore, examine convergence but at the same time pay attention to whether any nystagmus appears, by bringing the fixation target to 10–15 cm from the eyes. Absence of convergence is common after the age of 60 but in a younger person without a history of squint it can indicate a midbrain lesion.

Pursuit

Pursuit, or following movements, allows us clear vision of small objects moving slowly. Perfect pursuit is when the velocity of the eye matches that of the moving object. Young normal subjects pursue pretty well up to velocities of 40 deg/s (video clips 02.05 and 02.06). When the target moves faster the eye loses the target and, in order to catch up with it, puts in small *saccades*. These 'catch-up' saccades are visible to the clinician as a sudden, brisk movement towards the target.

When is pursuit abnormal? When pursuing a slowly moving target, the patient puts in too many catch-up saccades. The latter gives a 'broken up' or 'cogwheel' appearance to the pursuit movements. You must be sure that the patient is cooperating and attentive; use novel targets if he/she is not, such as a banknote or your keyring, and encourage him/her verbally. The target must move slowly, say taking 4–5 seconds to travel from 30 degrees right to 30 degrees left (or up–down) (video clips 02.05 and 02.06).

Clearly, following objects with the eyes is a function of the brain, not the labyrinth; thus, *the presence of pursuit abnormality indicates a central lesion* (video clip 02.23). Peripheral lesions have normal pursuit.

Pursuit abnormalities can be plane-specific (horizontal or vertical), in one direction (e.g. right or left), or generalised. Usually, unilateral pursuit abnormalities are on the same side as the CNS lesion. We will not discuss in full the anatomical basis of pursuit; it suffices to say that pursuit pathways are widespread in the CNS, particularly the cerebellum. This explains why pursuit is so sensitive to central lesions, but it also explains why *pursuit abnormalities are not site- or disease-specific*. The commonest causes of non-specific

Table 2.5 Sorting out pathological nystagmus

Type of nystagmus	Interpretation
Spontaneous nystagmus	
Horizontal (± torsional) with vertigo	Acute unilateral (usually peripheral) vestibular disorder
Horizontal pendular or jerky without vertigo or oscillopsia	Congenital nystagmus
Pendular, any direction with oscillopsia but no vertigo	Acquired pendular nystagmus (late multiple sclerosis vascular brainstem lesions)
Pure 'rotatory' (torsional)	Vestibular nuclear lesion
Upbeat	Midline brainstem lesion
Downbeat	Bilateral or mid line lesion of caudal cerebellum
With eccentric gaze	
In all directions of gaze	Cerebellar or brainstem gaze-evoked (gaze-paretic) nystagmus
Horizontal to one side only	Subacute peripheral vestibular disorder (first-degree nystagmus) or unilateral cerebellar lesion
Horizontal pendular or jerky without oscillopsia	Congenital, dampened in primary position
Horizontal on abducting eye with diminished adduction of fellow eye	Internuclear ophthalmoplegia due to midline brainstem lesion
Positional	
Torsional (± upbeat component), transient	BPPV of posterior canal
Horizontal to the ground in either lateral head position, transient	BPPV of horizontal canal (canalolithiasis)
Horizontal away from the ground in either lateral head position, long-lasting	BPPV of horizontal canal (cupulolithiasis) or central positional nystagmus
Downbeat, transient (± torsional component) with vertigo	BPPV of anterior canal
Downbeat, transient or persistent	Cerebellar lesion
Any other positional nystagmus	Suggestive of brainstem/cerebellar lesion (MRI!) or acute vestibular migraine
Head-shaking nystagmus	
Horizontal	Chronic unilateral peripheral vestibular disorder
Vertical	Brainsten or cerebellar lesion
With monocular fixation only	
Beating laterally away from the viewing eye	Latent nystagmus (variant of congenital nystagmus discovered during the cover test)

BPPV = benign paroxysmal positional vertigo

deteriorations of pursuit are old age and neuroactive drugs, so always interpret pursuit 'abnormalities' in the context of your patient's age and enquire about alcohol and psycho-pharmacological intake. *Pursuit after the age of 60 or 65 years is always broken up*; significant right–left asymmetries are still significant but this is not the case in the vertical plane.

Saccades

These are the eye movements that allow us to quickly move our eyes from one object to another. These refixation movements are fast (200–400 deg/s) and accurate. To investigate visually elicited saccades we provide the patient with two fixation targets, say two fingers or finger and pen, spaced ±30 degrees right–left or up–down (video clips 02.07 and 02.08). If you cannot see the patient's eyes well and need to open them up with your own fingers and thumb, you can ask the patient to refixate between your own ears. It is useful to verbally reinforce the patient by saying 'right ear – wait – left ear – wait – right ear' and so on.

There are two main abnormalities of saccades, both indicative of CNS disorder: saccadic inaccuracy (video clips 02.25 and 02.26) and saccadic slowing (02.27).

Inaccuracy occurs when the saccade is of the wrong size. It is easily detected because the eye makes two or more additional saccades in order to acquire the target. Hypometric saccades (the main saccade is smaller than it should be) are very common but non-specific; lesions anywhere in the CNS can provoke these (video clip 02.25). Hypermetric saccades, the equivalent of past pointing during the finger–nose test, indicate cerebellar disorder (video clip 02.26).

Slow saccades indicate brainstem (or eye muscle) disease, pontine for horizontal and midbrain for vertical saccades. When saccades are unequivocally slow, say 50% of their normal speed, this is very easy to detect as the eyes may take a second or more to acquire a new target (video clip 02.27). Detection of mild slowing needs training, but if you examine saccades in many of your patients you will quickly be able to pick up subtle abnormalities. This, as for pursuit, is of great practical value as it indicates CNS (or muscle) disease. Internuclear ophthalmoplegia manifests itself with slow or absent saccades of the adducting eye and concomitant nystagmus of the abducting eye. The lesion is located in the dorsal brainstem close to the midline and affects the medial longitudinal fasciculus which connects the abducens and the oculomotor nuclei (video clip 02.28).

Vestibular eye movements

Although confirmation of vestibular dysfunction often requires laboratory testing, clinical testing can provide important information in many cases. The majority of doctors seeing dizzy patients do not have their own vestibular laboratory and it is often better to rely on your own clinical examination than on unknown vestibular laboratories. Both the vestibulo-ocular reflex (VOR) and its suppression (VORS) can be examined in the clinic.

There are three specific clinical findings that have a reasonable degree of certainty: severe unilateral absence of vestibular function; severe bilateral absence of vestibular

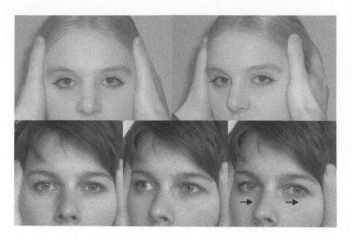

Figure 2.2 The head-impulse test. The examiner asks the patient to fixate an object straight ahead and then turns the head very rapidly to one side at a medium amplitude. A head turn to the patient's right side tests the right horizontal canal. The normal response (top row) consists of a compensatory eye movement to the left which occurs without delay. In a patient with loss of vestibular function on the right (bottom row) the eyes will first move in the direction of the head turn before a corrective, refixating saccade occurs in the opposite direction (i.e. towards your nose).

function; and abnormal VORS. The first two abnormalities are usually of a peripheral type, while the third type is always indicative of central disorder.

Severe unilateral vestibular hypofunction

This can be observed clinically. Think of the horizontal semicircular canals. We saw in Chapter 1 that head (nose) turning to the right activates the ipsilateral, right semicircular canal. This originates a slow-phase vestibular eye movement to the left, the VOR. If a lesion destroys the semicircular canal, the slow-phase VOR is weak and, for the eyes to remain on a fixation target, one or two saccades have to be put in. The fact that these saccades can be visible to the naked eye of an external observer constitutes the basis of the clinical manoeuvre called the 'head-thrust' or 'head-impulse' test (Figure 2.2).

The patient is seated, with the clinician facing him/her. You should be able to see the eyes well. The patient is told to fixate on, say, your nose or preferably on an object across the room. Patients must understand that they should keep their eyes on the target and that you are going to turn their head very fast. Then you apply a very fast, brisk movement to the right, then wait, then to the left and so on. In order to avoid the patient predicting the direction of your head stimulus, you can bring the patient's head back to midline slowly and then start again with the brisk stimulus (video clips 02.09 and 02.10). If during these stimuli the patient's eyes are consistently seen to generate a catch-up saccade towards the visual target, the labyrinth on the side you are turning the head to is not working (video clip 02.13).

If you are not confident with this test, an alternative is a simple cold- or ice-water caloric irrigation; the simplest version is the 20–20–20–20 test. The patient's head is lifted 20 degrees from supine, and 20 ml of water at 20 °C is irrigated over 20 seconds. The 'dead' ear will induce no dizziness or nystagmus, nor will it change a pre-existing spontaneous nystagmus. For less than total or subtotal vestibular lesions a formal caloric test is needed (see below).

In the same way that we can examine the VOR emanating from the horizontal semicircular canals with the head-impulse test, we can also assess the functioning of the four individual vertical canals. We will explain how to do this here in order to build up your understanding of how the vestibular system works, but the truth is that *selective* abnormalities of the superior or inferior canals are rare (you don't need to read this today if your first

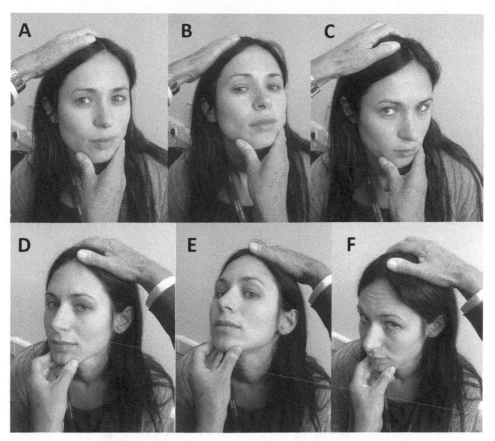

Figure 2.3 The head-impulse test for the vertical semicircular canals. With the head turned to the left (A) head movements along the sagittal plane of the body (not the sagittal plane of the head) stimulate the left posterior (B) and right anterior (C) semicircular canals. With the head turned to the right (D), backwards head movements stimulate the right posterior canal (E) while forward movements stimulate the left anterior (F) canal. Selective abnormalities in vertical canal function are very rare but in acute vestibular neuritis usually the horizontal and anterior (superior) canals are affected; hence in a right vestibular neuritis you would see the abnormality depicted in Figure 2.2 (bottom) and Figure 2.3 (C). If you are new to this field, get familiar with Figure 2.2 now and worry about Figure 2.3 later!

ever dizzy patient clinic starts tomorrow). First you must re-examine Figure 1.1 and its legend to remember that, with the head turned some 45 degrees to the left, flexion movements of the head activate the right anterior canal and extension movements of the head activate the left posterior canal, the so called RALP plane. With the head turned 45 degrees to the right, head flexion activates the left anterior and head extension the right posterior canals (the LARP plane). If you now examine Figure 2.3 you will see that, in a patient seated in front of you who is looking at your nose, these chin-down movements produce mostly vertical upwards eye movements whereas chin-up movements induce downwards eye movements. The head-impulse test for the LARP and RALP planes is therefore delivered by applying brief, fast movements in these planes and observing the patient's eye movements carefully. If a patient consistently introduces catch-up saccades to be able to keep fixating your nose during one of these four movements, it means that this particular canal is faulty. For example, in Figure 2.3, if a patient consistently puts in vertical catch-up saccades to look at your nose during movement 'E', she is likely to have right posterior canal hypofunction.

Severe bilateral absence of vestibular function

One should suspect bilateral vestibular failure when a patient reports bobbing oscillopsia or visual blurring when walking, running or riding in a vehicle, and when there is unsteadiness made worse in the dark (see page 141). All clinical manoeuvres able to detect bilateral vestibular failure are based on the physiological principle that the vestibulo-ocular reflex is responsible for gaze stability during head or whole-body movements. Here we will describe four procedures (Figures 2.2 and 2.4).

Head-impulse or head-thrust test

The head-thrust test described in the previous section will be positive during head thrusts both to the right and left (and also vertically) (video clip 02.14). Technically, this is decribed as a bilaterally positive or abnormal head-impulse test.

Head oscillation (doll's head-eye manoeuvre; video clips 02.11 and 02.12)

In most cases even a slower oscillation of the head, say once per second, usually reveals that the patient's eye movements are not actually smooth but cogwheeled, due to the presence of catch-up saccades.

Ophthalmoscopy

The ophthalmoscope can be used to observe small-amplitude nystagmus and assess the VOR. As for nystagmus, remember that you are seeing the retina which is at the back of the eye, so that a right- (or up-)beat nystagmus on funduscopy actually is a left- (or down-)beat nystagmus. Nystagmus due to a peripheral vestibular lesion can be small because VOR-suppression mechanisms keep it in check. In this case, plunging the viewing (non-examined) eye into the dark, by switching off all room lights or by asking the patient to cover the eye with a 'hollowed' hand, can make a peripheral vestibular nystagmus increase its amplitude. (NB: determining whether a nystagmus appears or increases on removing visual fixation, as just indicated with the ophthalmoscope, is the main use of Frenzel's glasses, described later.)

The VOR can be assessed with slow head oscillations whilst looking at the optic disc (Figure 2.4). The patient must keep visual fixation on a target across the room – and you must be out of the way (e.g. examine the patient's left eye with your left eye). With your free hand (right hand in Fig.2.4 top right) oscillate the patient's head slowly (1 Hz or less) and observe whether the disc remains fully stationary in space. If the disc 'jerks' this indicates either poor patient cooperation or catch-up saccades towards the visual target, indicative of a deficient VOR. (NB: the test can be positive unilaterally, in which case you can observe catch-up saccades only when the face turns in the direction of the damaged labyrinth.)

Dynamic visual acuity

This is probably the easiest way to clinically support the examination diagnosis of bilateral vestibular failure, particularly if your eye-movement examination skills are not great. Take a visual acuity chart (e.g. Snellen) at approximately the prescribed reading distance. Measure the baseline visual acuity which is the last line that the patient can read. For the purpose of VOR

Doll's head and head thrust

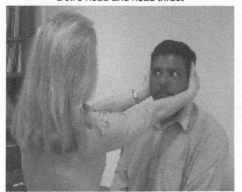

Dynamic funduscopy

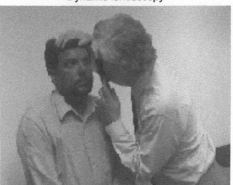

Dynamic visual acuity

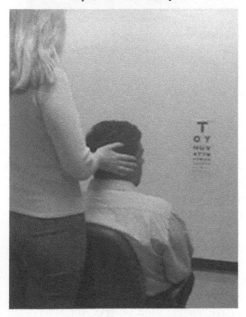

Figure 2.4 Clinical examination of the vestibulo-ocular reflex (VOR). Top left: oscillation of the head during doll's head-eye manoeuvre may show broken-up eye movements in cases of severe bilateral failure of the VOR. Single, fast, jerky movements of the head ('head-thrust test') are more effective, however, and can show unilateral defects of the VOR (see Figure 2.2). Top right: oscillation of the head during funduscopy may also reveal catch-up saccades (if they occur during nose rotation to the left, there is a left vestibular hypofunction). Bottom: measure binocular visual acuity in static conditions. Then oscillate the patient's head at about 1–2 Hz. Drops in visual acuity > 2 lines indicate severe bilateral vestibular failure.

testing this can be done binocularly. Then, whilst standing behind the patient, begin oscillating his/her head continuously at about 1–2 Hz and measure visual acuity during the head movement. Most normal people's visual acuity does not change but some may lose a line (i.e. from 6/6 they drop to 6/9). If they drop more than two lines (i.e. 6/6 to 6/12) there is a high suspicion that their VOR is not right. If they lose more than two lines (6/6 to 6/18 or worse) the patient has a very significant VOR failure. It is important to keep the head in continuous motion otherwise some patients get 'snaps' of the visual acuity chart and this may result in a false negativity.

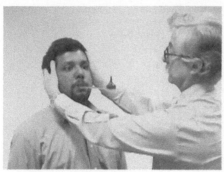
Head oscillation

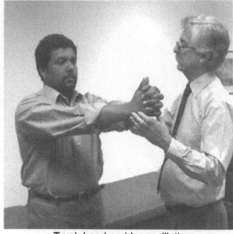
Trunk-head *en bloc* oscillation

Figure 2.5 Clinical examination of VOR suppression. The patient fixates on an object that is carried with his teeth (left) or on his own thumbs (right). The examiner should look carefully for the appearance of nystagmus elicited during head or trunk–head oscillation (abnormal or broken VOR suppression), which indicates a CNS disorder.

Abnormal VOR suppression

This is examined by having the patient fixating an object that moves *en bloc* with the head. The patient can look at his/her thumbs pointing up whilst the whole torso and head oscillate from side to side (Figure 2.5) (video clip 02.15) or look at a target attached at the end of a tongue depressor or a ruler carried by his/her teeth whilst only the head is oscillated at about 0.5 Hz or less. Normally the eyes should remain steadily fixed on the target; if significant nystagmus or asymmetric nystagmus is noticed then the patient has abnormal VOR suppression (video clip 02.24). This is an important central sign with a probable identical meaning to abnormal pursuit. Indeed, one should think of the VOR suppression situation as a 'head free' pursuit, like following the tennis ball with your eyes and head when watching a match. Abnormalities are co-directional, so that a patient with a right parietal or right cerebellar lesion will have abnormal pursuit or VOR suppression during target movement to the right. Similarly, as with pursuit, patients with peripheral vestibular lesions have normal VOR suppression.

Positional manoeuvres

The examination of positional vertigo and nystagmus is an essential step in the diagnosis of the dizzy patient (video clips 02.16–02.20). Benign paroxysmal positional vertigo is one the most common causes of vertigo and it is easily treatable, but it can be diagnosed only with positional testing. The topic is covered specifically in Chapter 5. Whilst BPPV has a specific set of symptoms, it is difficult to think of a particular dizzy patient in whom the positional manoeuvre is not worth doing. This is so because even patients with histories typical for other disorders (Ménière's disease, migraine, vestibular neuritis) may have developed secondary BPPV on a labyrinth damaged by the underlying disease. Even when you are not able to treat some of these underlying conditions successfully, you might be able to treat the BPPV. Similarly, patients with central disorders such as cerebellar degenerations or ischaemic brain disease often have central positional nystagmus, typically positional

A: Conventional Hallpike

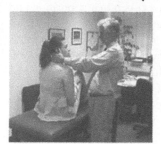

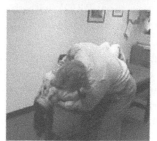

B: Modified Hallpike

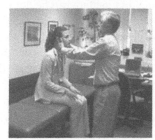

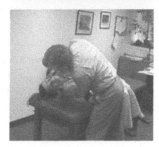

Figure 2.6 Conventional and modified Hallpike manoeuvre. A: shows the conventional positional Hallpike manoeuvre, examining for right-sided posterior canal BPPV. B: modified, 'sideways' variant Hallpike procedure. Note the similar final head position achieved with both procedures. When examining for BPPV these manoeuvres should be conducted fairly briskly. C: the typical nystagmus in right-sided posterior canal BPPV; torsional nystagmus beating to the undermost ear (in this case right) with a small upbeat component (see video clip 05.01).

C: 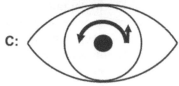 Right-beating torsional nystagmus in BPPV

downbeat nystagmus (video clip 05.12 and 05.13). The finding of a positional nystagmus in a patient with CNS disease indicates that part of the patient's balance symptoms are due to central vestibular dysfunction.

The purpose of conducting a positional manoeuvre is to try to elicit vertigo and nystagmus, but vertigo is unpleasant. The patient should be made aware that despite modern technology this is the only way to make a diagnosis of a perfectly treatable condition such as BPPV. During the positional manoeuvre, and regardless of whether there is vertigo or not, the examiner should carefully observe the patient's eyes. In order to fulfil this purpose the following practical measures can be taken:

1. Patients should be warned beforehand that, even if they feel vertiginous, they should look straight ahead at one point on the examiner's face (i.e. the nose or bridge of the nose). If the eyes are not in primary gaze or wandering around, the observation of the nystagmus is more difficult.
2. At least one eye of the patient can be easily helped to stay wide open by one of the free hands of the examiner, as shown in video clips 02.16–02.19 and in Figure 2.6.
3. Keep the patient in the ear-down position for a few seconds. Some patients with BPPV show extremely long latencies, exceptionally up to 15–20 seconds. If the suspicion of BPPV is strong one should wait this long but most cases of BPPV have latencies of 4–5 seconds.

There are no excuses for not conducting a positional manoeuvre. However, two of the most commonly heard excuses are 'the couch in my room is placed awkwardly to do a Hallpike,

I just cannot get the patient's head to hang off the couch' and 'we haven't got Frenzel's glasses in our clinic'. Wrong! A positional manoeuvre can be done with a couch in any position and Frenzel's glasses are definitely *not* required for positional nystagmus. Figure 2.6 shows both the conventional Hallpike manoeuvre with the classical head-hanging position and a recommended alternative to the procedure when, for instance, the couch is placed between walls or cupboards. Comparison of these pictures shows that the final head position achieved is very similar. As to the use of Frenzel's glasses remember that the classical descriptions of BPPV by Dix and Hallpike were carried out without Frenzel's glasses!

What can we expect to see during a Hallpike or 'variant Hallpike' manoeuvre? The most common form of positional nystagmus is BPPV of the posterior canal. During a left-ear-down head-hanging position one triggers a left posterior canal BPPV, with the main component of the nystagmus being torsional (or rotatory) beating clockwise from the observer point of view. This means that the top ('north pole') of the patient's eye beats towards the patient's left shoulder. Technically speaking it is left-beating torsional nystagmus, as expected from activation of the left posterior canal. A secondary upbeat component of nystagmus is often observed which is synchronous with the torsional beat. The nystagmus is often accompanied by intense vertigo and by the patient's attempt to close the eyes or to sit up – which the doctor will have hopefully instructed him/her in advance to resist. The characteristics of posterior canal BPPV are the presence of latency, as mentioned above, the short duration of the nystagmus and its decline if one were to repeat the manoeuvre. The positional manoeuvre should be conducted on both sides, particularly if no nystagmus is observed on the first side. On confirmation of the diagnosis, you should proceed directly to the treatment with particle repositioning manoeuvres like the Epley or Semont manoeuvre (Chapter 5; video clips 05.02–05.05).

Variants of BPPV involving the horizontal and anterior semicircular canal do exist but we would advise at this stage that if the positional manoeuvre provokes any nystagmus different to the one described above, particularly up- or downbeat nystagmus, you consider the possibility that your patient may have a CNS disorder. For further details on positional vertigo, nystagmus and its treatment see Chapter 5.

Frenzel's glasses

The availability of Frenzel's glasses in ENT or neurology clinics varies from country to country and, within a country, from hospital to hospital. Essentially, Frenzel's glasses are goggles fitted with positive (+) lenses of approximately 10–12 diopters (i.e. a magnifying glass). The goggles are illuminated inside, so that an observer can see the patient's eyes enlarged and clearly (Figure 2.7). Since the glasses are close to the patient's eyes, he/she has completely blurred vision and therefore cannot visually fixate on any object. As a consequence, Frenzel's glasses are an excellent way to observe the patient's eyes in the absence of optic fixation. Or to put it the other way round, you would use Frenzel's glasses when you suspect that a patient may have nystagmus but you cannot see it by naked eye because it may be suppressed by visual fixation.

That is the general principle, but what are the specific uses of Frenzel's glasses?

• In peripheral unilateral vestibular lesions, Frenzel's glasses may make a nystagmus increase in amplitude appear or – this is the main application of Frenzel's glasses (video clip 03.01). In contrast, the nystagmus in central lesions does not increase with Frenzel's

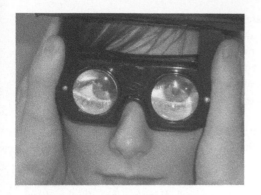

Figure 2.7 Frenzel's glasses. The high optic magnification impedes the patient fixating any object (particularly if the room is dimly lit). A nystagmus which appears or enhances during Frenzel's glasses observation is likely to be of peripheral vestibular origin. See video clip 03.01.

glasses and in congenital nystagmus it may even reduce in size or stop beating altogether.

- If in a patient with a suspected unilateral peripheral lesion no nystagmus is observed by direct and Frenzel's-glasses observation, vigorously shaking the head horizontally (no–no) 20 times may make the nystagmus reappear under Frenzel's observation. (video clip 03.01)
- Positional manoeuvres do not need to be done with Frenzel's glasses routinely. The nystagmus in posterior canal BPPV (Table 5.1), by far the most common positional nystagmus in the clinic, is very strong and is mostly torsional – a plane in which visual suppression is not very effective. Similarly, patients with central positional nystagmus have, in parallel, defective VOR suppression and therefore vision is usually incapable of suppressing a positional nystagmus. Therefore, only in some patients with a weak peripheral BPPV (particularly horizontal canal cupulo-lithiasis), and in patients with central positional vertigo with preserved VOR suppression, may Frenzel's glasses reveal a nystagmus that is otherwise not visible by naked-eye observation. Since these situations are truly exceptional we cannot recommend the routine use of Frenzel's glasses during the positional manoeuvre. Instead we use them when the two situations mentioned above are suspected.

Posture and gait

Examination of posture and gait can shed useful light in the diagnosis of the dizzy patient but, relatively speaking, it is less important than eye movements or the positional man-oeuvre. Gait unsteadiness is associated with a wide range of disorders, but if it has never been associated with vertigo, dizziness, oscillopsia or hearing disorder it is unlikely to be due to vestibular disease.

Observation of *stance* will reveal a broadening of the base of support in diffuse vascular disease, frontal lesions, cerebellar lesions, sensory ataxia, acute or bilateral vestibular lesions and patients with a cautious gait. Lateropulsion can be seen in acute unilateral peripheral vestibular lesions and in lateralised brainstem–cerebellar lesions. Midline cerebellar–brainstem lesions can show retropulsion. Minor degrees of unsteadiness can be brought about by asking the patient to put his/her feet together or in the heel-to-toe position.

The *Romberg test* is positive in patients with dorsal-column or severe afferent poly-neuropathy (video clip 07.01). A positive Romberg means that the patient shows a tendency to actually fall after closing his eyes – unlike normal subjects and almost all patients with balance problems who show a small to moderate increase in body sway on eye closure. Only in the acute phase of a peripheral vestibular disorder will the Romberg test be positive, usually with an ipsilesional fall. Of practical note, anyone who can stand on either foot unaided, with eyes closed, is unlikely to have any objective postural balance problem. The Romberg test can be sensitised with regard to unilateral vestibular hypofunction by asking the patient to stand in the tandem (heel-to-toe) position; patients with significant hypofunction tend to lean ipsilesionally.

Postural reflexes are examined by gently pushing and pulling the upper trunk. This can be done while standing behind the patient so he/she cannot anticipate the precise timing and direction of the push to the shoulders (forwards or backwards). Vestibular patients may be unsteady but the overall pattern of the response is preserved. For this reason these reflexes do not need to be investigated in the conventional dizzy patient. In the elderly, with fear of falling or a cautious gait, trunk pushes trigger a startle, a panic-like response. The main abnormality, absence of these responses, occurs in parkinsonian syndromes, idiopathic or vascular, where patients may fall 'as a log' (video clips 02.29 and 07.05).

It is useful, however, to see your dizzy patient walk first with eyes open and then with eyes closed. A number of peripheral and central neurological disorders can be detected during *eyes-open gait*; but, as far as vestibular disease is concerned, most patients walk normally, unless in an acute, vertiginous stage. Some patients with balance complaints deploy a cautious or rather overcautious gait. The arms of a patient with a cautious gait reach out as if expecting a fall, and he/she steps with apparently unnecessary care, giving the appearance of 'walking on ice'. Although a cautious gait can be part of a psychogenic gait disorder it can be triggered by a vestibular, vascular or falling episode. Sometimes this is the only finding in elderly patients.

Walking in a straight line with eyes closed can reveal a previously unsuspected degree of unsteadiness or a cautious gait in patients with bilateral loss of vestibular function. In somatosensory ataxia, as in tabes dorsalis or severe polyneuropathies, this task is often impossible. In unilateral vestibular lesions, particularly in the acute stage, patients veer in the same direction as the lesion. In the *Unterberger test*, instead of walking along, the patient is asked to walk 50 steps on the spot with eyes closed (Figure 2.8). In unilateral vestibular lesions the patient turns more than 60° towards the hypoactive side. It is helpful to ask the patient to keep the arms and index fingers pointing forwards towards the examiner's index fingers; this allows a more precise assessment of the degree and consistency of turning. It is useful to repeat the Unterberger test, looking for consistency in the patient's deviation, and whether there is a congruent gait deviation when walking with eyes closed. As the Unterberger test is somewhat time-consuming, and because there are other tests to detect unilateral vestibular hypofunction clinically, it is less frequently used nowadays.

If at this stage you have detected what appears to be abnormal tone, strength or coordination of the locomotor muscles, a formal neurological examination is called for, by yourself or a specialist. This will not be dealt with here, but *weakness of the legs* can be documented by asking the patient to stand/walk on tiptoes and heels, crouch and rise. Identification of weakness of the ankle extensors is paramount as these muscles are responsible for toe clearance during the swing phase of the gait cycle. The *tendon jerks* will be exaggerated in pyramidal tract disease but depressed or absent in weakness due to root or peripheral nerve disease; extensor cutaneous plantar responses (Babinski sign) can be found in pyramidal tract lesions. *Somatosensory function* can be assessed with pin-prick stimuli, tuning fork and joint position sense in the lower limbs. If the reason for your patient's

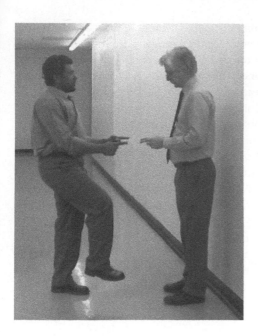

Figure 2.8 The 'stepping on the spot' or **Unterberger test.** The patient walks with eyes closed on the spot while the examiner watches for reproducible rotation to one side which indicates the side of vestibular hypofunction.

unsteadiness is that large fibres carrying proprioceptive input are involved, the ankle and sometimes patella jerks will be absent and the Romberg test will be positive.

It is important to keep in mind the unabated weight of the clinical neurological examination in the assessment of balance and gait disorders. Observation of gait, postural reflexes and the Romberg test followed, if appropriate, by a quick examination of lower limb power, coordination, reflexes and tuning fork are likely to help more than posturography (see below). Normal CT and MRI scans are very valuable but do not exclude neurological disease (e.g. Parkinson's), and posturography findings usually lack topographical and aetiological specificity. Functional (psychogenic) disorders can be diagnosed on the basis of an inconsistent or theatrical gait pattern, in a patient with otherwise essentially normal findings.

Clinical assessment of hearing

Hearing should be assessed clinically in all dizzy patients. All patients should be directly asked about hearing loss or tinnitus. Your chances of encountering positive findings on examination are higher in the presence of unilateral symptoms, but you must examine the external auditory canal with an otoscope to make sure that impacted wax is not the cause of the deafness. Check whether there is an asymmetry of hearing with the ticking of a watch, rubbing your thumb and fingers or muttering words to each ear. For the thumb–finger rubbing test, start from a distance with your arm fully stretched and come in towards the patient's ear. Compare the distance at which the patient says 'Yes, I can hear it' for each ear.

If you identify a hearing loss (uni- or bilateral) try to ascertain whether it is conductive (middle or outer ear) or sensorineural (cochlear or eighth nerve – brainstem lesions rarely produce unilateral hearing loss). This is done with tuning forks, but beware that some low-frequency tuning forks (64 or 128 Hz), as used for the neurological examination of vibration sense, can produce unreliable results. For the *Rinne test*, place the foot of the vibrating tuning fork on the mastoid (bone conduction) and then place the prongs in front of the auditory meatus (air conduction); ask the patient which one is louder. Normally (positive Rinne) air conduction is louder, and this pattern is retained in a sensorineural hearing loss. If bone conduction is louder (negative Rinne) the hearing loss is conductive; caution should be exercised as a profound unilateral sensorineural hearing loss can produce a false-negative Rinne due to the fact that the sound will be bone-perceived by the contralateral good ear.

In the *Weber test*, the foot or base of the tuning fork is placed on the vertex. The patient is asked if the sound stays in the middle (top) of the head or whether it is louder in either ear. If it is louder in the deaf ear, the hearing loss is conductive. In severe unilateral sensorineural deafness the patient will be able to report the sound only in the good ear. If a dizzy patient reports deafness, particularly in one ear, formal audiological tests should be arranged.

Conductive hearing loss potentially relevant to dizziness can be seen in some cases of otosclerosis or in destructive middle-ear disease (e.g. a cholesteatoma). However, it is sensorineural loss that is normally relevant to dizziness, e.g. ototoxicity, labyrinthine hydrops (e.g. Ménière's disease) and vascular, inflammatory or tumoural processes of the labyrinth or eighth nerve.

Orthostatic blood pressure

Orthostatic hypotension is often suggested by the history but requires measurement of orthostatic blood pressure for confirmation. The first blood pressure is assessed in the supine position after a few minutes of rest. The patient is then asked to stand up for repeated measurements in the upright position for three minutes. A fall of at least 20 mmHg in systolic blood pressure or at least 10 mmHg in diastolic blood pressure is regarded as relevant. Orthostatic hypotension can go unrecognised when measurements are made at times that do not correspond to the patient's usual symptomatic periods, which are often in the morning or after meals.

Laboratory examinations

If the cause of the dizziness in a patient is not suspected or presumed from the history and examination, it is unlikely that laboratory investigations will make it clear. Investigations can, however, provide strong support for or against certain presumed diagnoses. In this section our aim is that you learn which tests are available, their physiological basis, how they can help you in reaching a diagnosis and when you need them.

We will cover the tests in an approximate order of both general availability and usefulness. Many more audiometric and vestibular tests than are mentioned here are available, but because they are for specialised neuro-otologists and not widely available, they will not be discussed here. (See 'Further reading', page 183.)

Pure-tone audiogram

Any dizzy patient who complains of tinnitus, hearing loss or aural pressure should undergo pure-tone audiometry. These symptoms are more significant if they are unilateral as presbiacusis or Eustachian tube dysfunction account for a large majority of aural and hearing symptoms. A pure-tone audiogram measures hearing thresholds at different frequencies; this can be performed via normal air conduction or by bone conduction and in this way conductive and sensorineural hearing loss (SNHL) can be differentiated.

Sensorineural hearing loss in patients with dizziness is expected in Ménière's disease and in inflammatory, neoplastic and vascular disorders of the labyrinth or the eighth nerve.

In Ménière's disease, at least initially, the hearing loss is prominent at low frequencies. As in other labyrinthine lesions, patients have recruitment in the hypoacousic ear, meaning that the gap between hearing thresholds and discomfort elicited by loud sounds is narrower than normal. The discomfort levels can be measured subjectively, delivering loud sounds with the audiometer, or objectively measuring stapedial reflex thresholds.

Brainstem auditory-evoked potentials will not be discussed in detail here. Many of these audiological tests were developed with acoustic neuromas and demyelination in mind, but the refinement and wide availability of imaging procedures have superseded these. As a rule of thumb, any patient with a unilateral or significantly asymmetrical sensorineural hearing loss should have an MRI with good views of the cerebellopontine angle to rule out a space-occupying lesion. Nevertheless, auditory-evoked potentials retain their screening power and a patient with normal potentials is very unlikely to have an acoustic neuroma.

Caloric testing

This is one of the most useful 'laboratory' tests in the assessment of dizzy patients. Although it is relatively 'low tech', it is the only simple test that gives you mono-aural information and it has stood the test of time. Make sure first that there is no gross middle-ear disease or wax precluding the irrigation!

In all variants of the test the patient's head has to be placed 20–30 degrees up from horizontal (or 60 degrees down from vertical) so that the horizontal semicircular canals are oriented vertically. In its simplest form, irrigating with a few millilitres of ice-water, one ear at a time, and timing the duration of nystagmus will be enough to tell you whether a patient has a severe asymmetry of vestibular function. One step up from this is the 20–20–20 test: irrigation with water at 20 °C, delivered with a 20 ml syringe over 20 seconds. The observer times the duration of the irrigation-induced nystagmus.

A test adopted universally, standardised by Fitzgerald and Hallpike, uses water at two different temperatures, 30 and 44 °C (i.e. 7 degrees below and above body temperature). Each ear is irrigated for 40 seconds, with a rest of approximately 5 minutes between them. In this bi-thermal form, the test not only informs about loss of response from one ear ('canal paresis') but also about symmetry, or lack of it, in the vestibulo-ocular reflex ('directional preponderance'). A third important abnormality is the patient with little or no nystagmic response from either ear ('bilateral loss of vestibular function'). Normally, vestibular responses are recorded by electro-oculography (or 'nystagmography') or video-oculography (Figure 2.9), but timing nystagmus duration by naked eye is also a valid measurement. We do not provide further information on this test here because it is specialist territory; this can be found under 'Further reading'.

When do you need this test in your patient, as a must? Again, the answer is relative to whether you will be practising at a specialist or non-specialist level. As a non-specialist, you do need caloric test results when the clinical picture in your patient is not typical of any established disorder. In this case a significant canal paresis or directional preponderance will indicate that the patient does suffer from a vestibular disorder. Put another way, if the

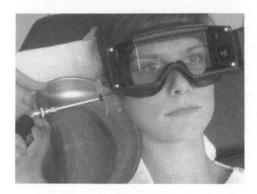

Figure 2.9 Caloric test. Note that during testing, the video-oculography mask is covered in order to record eye movements in the dark. Otherwise, visual fixation would suppress vestibular nystagmus to a certain degree.

clinical picture is typical of BPPV, vestibular neuritis, Ménière's disease (with audiometric confirmation), psychogenic dizziness or brainstem stroke (e.g. Wallenberg syndrome), you do not really need a caloric test. As a specialist interested in dizziness you will want somehow to document vestibular function in most of your patients.

Rotational tests and video head-impulse test (vHIT)

Rotating chair tests stimulate the vestibular system physiologically, but it is difficult to know which vestibular apparatus, right or left, is responsible for an abnormality. Therefore there are only two possible abnormalities, either asymmetry (or directional preponderance) or bilateral reduction of vestibular function. As in caloric testing, assessment is normally based on oculography.

An interesting new development of the last few years is the emergence of systems that record the head and eye movements during manually delivered head impulses, as described above, page 36 ('Vestibular eye movement'; Figure 2.2; video clips 2.09, 2.10 and 2.13). This allows documentation of the slow-phase eye movement and the 'catch-up saccade' which can enhance the sensitivity of the clinical head-impulse test – the video head-impulse test or vHIT. There are several commercially available systems and some of them can examine all six semicircular canals. These systems are very helpful and easy to use but we do not think that they replace caloric testing.

Video-oculography (VOG), videonystagmography (VNG), electronystagmography (ENG) and electro-oculography (EOG)

A clinician can view all these terms as essentially similar techniques for recording eye movements. These procedures can be applied for recording of nystagmus during caloric or rotational responses, and many systems are commercially available. In practice, when a clinician requests a VOG or an ENG other tests are included, essentially an assessment of the eye movements described above in the clinical examination section.

The clinician should be aware that many VOG reports (often produced by technicians) suggest a 'central vestibular disorder' not on the basis of the caloric or rotational findings but on abnormalities of pursuit, saccades or optokinetic nystagmus. Since these non-vestibular oculomotor abnormalities may be due to attentional factors or psychoactive drugs, the clinician should rely more on his/her own oculomotor examination and clinical judgement than on a VOG report. The situation is even worse for positional or neck-

Video 02.29 – Normal postural reflexes
Normal postural reactions (or reflexes) in a healthy young subject: trunk pushes and pulls elicit a quick, single, protective stepping response that fully stabilises the body. Usually the pushes are delivered from behind so the patient cannot predict the direction of the stimulus. This also reassures and protects the patient in case they should fall backwards. When testing patients or elderly people an assistant should stand in front of the patient (ready to catch). If the patients are not very unsteady or frail, they can face a wall, corner of the room (video clip) or couch so that they may use their arms to arrest a possible fall. This examination is always conducted with the eyes open.

rotation induced nystagmus since there are no norms for these procedures. If you think your patient may have a positional nystagmus you must do a *Hallpike manoeuvre*, not request an eye-movement recording.

A routine VOG also includes a search for spontaneous and gaze-evoked nystagmus. Since oculography can be carried out in the dark, this does add useful information normally not available to the clinician unless he/she is furnished with an infrared viewer or Frenzel's glasses. If a nystagmus appears on removal of fixation, either by VOG, infrared viewing in the dark (available on some phone apps) or Frenzel's glasses, this is strong evidence in favour of a vestibular disorder, usually of a peripheral type. Finally, video cameras or smartphones can be an excellent way of documenting an eye-movement abnormality – and patients with episodic disorders can get their own eyes videoed at home.

In summary, if the VOG or caloric test's report states that there is a significant canal paresis and/or nystagmus in the dark, take that as good evidence in favour of a peripheral vestibular disorder. If the report says that there is significant directional preponderance (or asymmetry of the VOR) that is good evidence in favour of vestibular asymmetry, the origin of which will have to be ascertained by the clinical and laboratory context. If the report suggests evidence of a 'central vestibular disorder', try to see what this evidence is. If it is abnormalities of saccades, pursuit or VOR suppression, try to confirm these findings with your own clinical examination, or with that of a colleague with eye-movement expertise (e.g. neurologist or neuro-ophthalmologist).

Other tests such as vestibular-evoked myogenic potentials (VEMPs) or posturography are not essential for diagnosis of the common balance or dizziness problems.

Separating peripheral from central vestibular lesions

Tables 2.6 and 2.7 attempt to summarise the features which allow separation between peripheral and central vestibular lesions. Essentially, unilateral peripheral vestibular lesions would in the acute stage produce a tendency to fall ipsilesionally and show a horizontal or horizontal–torsional nystagmus beating contralesionally. (If you think of the slow phase, which is what matters, both the body and the eyes drift towards the side of the lesion.) As the process of vestibular compensation gets under way, the nystagmus and unsteadiness are suppressed. Apart from the initial nystagmus and a possible positive head-thrust test, the remainder of the eye movements – such as VOR suppression, pursuit and saccades – remain normal throughout. Any departure from this scheme may indicate a central disorder.

In spite of the traditional separation between peripheral and central vestibular signs, we must emphasise that classification of the lesion as peripheral or central is only one stage in the diagnostic process. The final aim is to make a specific diagnosis, which in some cases

Table 2.6 Guide for peripheral versus central vestibular disorders

	Peripheral	Central
CNS exam/symptoms	–	+/+++
Auditory exam/symptoms	Frequently +	Usually –
Unsteadiness:		
acute	+++	+++
chronic	+/–	+++
Eye-movements	Normal	Usually abnormal
Vertigo:		
acute	+++	++
chronic	+/–	+/–

CNS = central nervous system

Table 2.7 Guide for peripheral versus central nystagmus

	Peripheral	Central
Plane[a]	Horizontal, or horizontal > torsional	Any
Amplitude:		
acute	++	++/+++
chronic	+/–	++/+++
Fixation removal[b]	Appears/enhances	Variable
Waveform[c]	Rectilinear[c]	Exponential[c], pendular

[a] This table is for *spontaneous* nystagmus since peripheral *positional* nystagmus, as in BPPV, is predominantly torsional.
[b] By oculography, Frenzel's glasses, infrared viewer or funduscopy in the dark.
[c] By oculography only (specialist procedure), it refers to the slow component of a jerk nystagmus.

such as migraine (page 71) and vascular disease (page 64) often combine peripheral and central vestibular components.

Imaging procedures in dizzy patients

A main reason to request neuroradiological investigations in patients with dizziness and vertigo is to rule out or confirm the presence of a structural lesion (see Table 2.8). However, in view of the fact that the most frequent causes of vertigo do not produce abnormal images (e.g. vestibular neuritis, migraine, BPPV and Ménière's disease), the vast majority of brain scans in dizzy patients are negative. With this in mind physicians should exercise restraint and not request imaging in all dizzy patients. Not only is this onerous for the public and private medicine sectors, it is also often a source of additional worry for the patient when 'normal variants', 'unrelated findings', 'benign cysts' and 'age-related changes' are reported. It follows that we should try to define which patients deserve a scan, although this should be

Table 2.8 Indications for brain scanning in dizzy patients

Reason for scanning	Expected finding/diagnosis	Exceptions (scan not imperative)
V, VI, VII, limb symptoms	Brainstem disease (stroke, multiple sclerosis)	
Spontaneous nystagmus	Central vestibular disorder (brainstem or cerebellar disease)	Acute peripheral disorder, congenital nystagmus
Atypical positional nystagmus	Central vestibular disorder	
Oscillopsia	Central vestibular disorder	Absent vestibular function of known cause (e.g. ototoxicity)
Gait disorder	Ischaemic disease, degenerative disorders, hydrocephalus, subdural haematoma, cerebellar atrophy, Arnold–Chiari malformation, cord compression	Typical idiopathic Parkinson's disease Peripheral neuropathy
Unilateral hearing symptoms	Acoustic neuroma	Audiogram and brainstem auditory potentials normal

counterbalanced with the fact that many patients with long-term or frightening symptoms believe that 'there's something wrong' with their brain. Physicians will have to be flexible and accept that, in a few cases, some patients will have to be scanned solely for the purpose of reassurance.

The most important criterion for requesting imaging procedures is the presence of symptoms or signs indicating cranial nerve or CNS disorder. In the patient with vertigo the more prominent are diplopia, facial tingling, numbness or weakness, unilateral tinnitus or hearing loss, limb incoordination, weakness or sensory symptoms.

The presence of spontaneous nystagmus requires imaging, particularly if it can be identified as central (e.g. down- or upbeat, torsional, gaze-paretic, pendular). Exceptions to this rule would be: (a) the patient with an acute peripheral vestibular cause (e.g. vestibular neuritis) or caught in the middle of a known recurrence such as migraine or Ménière's disease; and (b) congenital nystagmus, either because this is known to pre-exist, because of the lack of visuo-vestibular symptoms, or if confirmed by pathognomonic nystagmus waveforms on oculography.

Positional nystagmus does not require imaging if the clinical course and positional findings are typical of posterior canal or horizontal canal BPPV (see Chapter 5). Persistent positional nystagmus (i.e. lack of adaptation) may indicate the rarer cupulolithiasis as opposed to canalolithiasis, but it could equally indicate a central disorder and therefore it would be safer to obtain an MRI scan.

Patients with oscillopsia are also likely to require a brain scan – Table 2.4 shows that the majority of causes of oscillopsia are central disorders. The exception would be patients with movement-provoked oscillopsia, when you have good clinical or laboratory evidence that the cause of the oscillopsia is a severe reduction in vestibular function, e.g. a patient with a bilaterally positive head-thrust test following gentamicin intoxication.

It is difficult to generalise on the need for brain scans in patients with gait disorders. Typical cases of idiopathic Parkinson's disease do not need a brain scan, which will usually be normal. Patients with focal symptoms or findings, eye-movement disorder, cognitive features, a past medical history of relevance (e.g. vascular risk factors, head injury, malignancy, autoimmune disease, positive family history) should be scanned. Patients with symptoms or findings suggestive of a spinal cord level (spastic paraparesis, sensory level, bladder dysfunction) should have the spine MRI-scanned urgently, because gait unsteadiness can turn into permanent paraplegia very quickly when the cause is a spinal cord compression.

Acoustic neuromas

One of the specific worries in neuro-otology is missing an acoustic neuroma (vestibular schwannoma) or other cerebellopontine space-occupying lesion. Whilst this is understandable, a few comments are warranted:

1. Although balance symptoms can occur these are rare. The vast majority of acoustic neuromas present with auditory symptoms, typically unilateral tinnitus and progressive hearing loss.
2. Acoustic neuromas are not infrequently seen in MRI scans as unrelated findings.
3. The growth rate of acoustic neuromas is quite slow, so that in many patients, particularly the elderly or infirm, a follow-up scan and audiometry at 6–12 months is recommended rather than immediate surgery.

Although MRI is the most specific and sensitive procedure for acoustic neuromas and other cerebellopontine-angle lesions, it is expensive as a screening procedure. In fact, only approximately 10–20% of patients with suspected retrocochlear disorders will have a positive scan, so audiometric protocols are constantly devised as screening protocols. In principle, a patient with a normal audiogram and a normal brainstem auditory-evoked potential is very unlikely to have an acoustic neuroma. In contrast, patients with a unilateral (or asymmetric) hearing loss of 20 dB or more in two contiguous frequencies, or with a unilateral abnormality of brainstem potentials, should be MRI-scanned. Of course, the presence of additional neurological findings indicative of cerebellopontine-angle occupation, such as an abnormal corneal reflex or other abnormalities of nerves V, VI and VII, necessitate MRI investigation.

Finally, what scan should be obtained? If the cause of concern is a cerebellopontine tumour or any other posterior fossa disorder, an MRI should be requested. CT scans have poor resolution and suffer from many artefacts in the posterior fossa. However if a bony lesion is suspected, petrous bone fractures or superior canal dehiscence (Chapter 4), a CT scan is indicated.

Chapter 3

A single episode of prolonged vertigo

This chapter is written from the perspective of primary care and emergency doctors who actually see patients with a first episode of acute vertigo. This clinical presentation is also called *acute vestibular syndrome*, particularly when vertigo is accompanied by nausea, vomiting and imbalance. In this situation, decision-making is both difficult and critical because there is no previous diagnosis to rely on and benign conditions such as vestibular neuritis and vestibular migraine have to be separated from serious disorders such as brainstem or cerebellar stroke. Table 3.1 provides an overview.

Table 3.1 Single episode of prolonged vertigo: diagnoses with key features

Disorder	Key features
Vestibular neuritis (page 54)	Acute onset of vertigo, nausea and imbalance Contralesional spontaneous nystagmus, ipsilesional VOR failure (positive head-impulse test), falls towards affected side Improvement over days to weeks
Acute brainstem or cerebellar lesion (e.g. stroke, demyelination) (page 60)	Vertigo with brainstem or cerebellar signs Variable time course MRI usually shows lesion affecting central vestibular pathways
Herpes zoster oticus (page 66)	Acute unilateral vestibular loss with facial palsy and one or more of the following: ear pain, vesicular rash, hearing loss, tinnitus, meningitis
First attack of vestibular migraine (page 66)	Acute vertigo, may last hours or days Mostly central types of vestibular nystagmus and ataxia History of migraine and often migraine symptoms during attack
First attack of BPPV (page 67)	Repetitive brief vertigo attacks may be interpreted as a single prolonged attack. Triggered by head positioning, positive Hallpike manoeuvre
First attack of Ménière's disease (page 67)	Vertigo lasting hours, may be isolated symptom in early Ménière's disease Otherwise, associated hearing loss, tinnitus and aural fullness
Other causes (page 67)	Labyrinthine infarction, perilymph fistula, bacterial labyrinthitis, drug/alcohol toxicity

VOR = vestibulo-ocular reflex; MRI = magnetic resonance imaging; BPPV = benign paroxysmal positional vertigo.

Vestibular neuritis

(Synonyms: vestibular neuronitis, viral neurolabyrinthitis, acute unilateral vestibular failure, acute unilateral peripheral vestibulopathy; see Table 3.2.)

Clinical features

With an annual incidence of at least 3.5 per 100,000 population, vestibular neuritis is the second most common peripheral vestibular disorder after benign paroxysmal positional vertigo (BPPV). Any hospital's emergency department will see several such patients per year. Vestibular neuritis starts acutely with intense vertigo, which persists for days and weeks. Some patients have a preceding respiratory tract infection and some experience warnings in the form of brief attacks of vertigo a day or two in advance. The vertigo reaches its maximum within minutes or hours and is associated with oscillopsia, nausea, vomiting and veering or falling to one side. Any head movement aggravates the vertigo so that patients prefer to lie still. Unable to walk, most patients reach the hospital on a stretcher with a sick bag placed next to them. Often, they are frightened by the experience of persisting vertigo and fears range from having a stroke to impending death.

Clinical examination within the first few days reveals the signs of acute unilateral vestibular failure (see below) – but nothing else:

- *Spontaneous nystagmus beating to the healthy ear.* The nystagmus is predominantly horizontal, but has also a torsional component with the upper pole of the eye beating to the healthy side. Its intensity is modified by direction of gaze and visual fixation: it increases when the patient looks in the direction of the fast nystagmus component or when visual fixation is removed by Frenzel's glasses, and it decreases when the patient looks in the opposite direction (Figure 3.1 and video clip 3.01). Admittedly however, one initially does not know which is the healthy or sick ear, given that vestibular neuritis does not induce auditory

Table 3.2 Vestibular neuritis: key features

History	Acute onset of vertigo, nausea, vomiting and veering to one side Spontaneous recovery over days or weeks
Clinical findings	Spontaneous nystagmus towards healthy ear, partly suppressed by visual fixation Pathological head-impulse test with rapid head rotation towards involved side, directional postural imbalance towards affected side
Pathophysiology	Probably viral/postviral infection of the vestibular nerve leading to sudden asymmetry of neural activity in the vestibular nuclei
Investigations	Caloric testing, vHIT or audiometry (not required in clear cases); MRI only when there are neurological abnormalities or in patients with vascular risk factors
Treatment	Exercise therapy promotes restoration of balance. Debate regarding use of oral steroids

MRI = magnetic resonance imaging; vHIT = video-based head-impulse test.

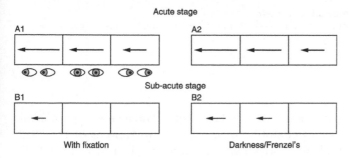

Figure 3.1 Nystagmus due to acute loss of vestibular function on the left (only the main, horizontal component is shown).
A: Acute stage (first day) with and without visual fixation. B: Subacute stage (after one week) with and without fixation. The size of the arrow symbolises nystagmus intensity. The figure illustrates three rules for peripheral vestibular nystagmus: (1) Nystagmus is partly suppressed by fixation and thus becomes more prominent in darkness or with Frenzel's glasses. (2) Nystagmus increases when the patient looks in the direction of the nystagmus fast phase and decreases in the opposite direction (Alexander's law). (3) Nystagmus intensity decreases in the course of time, i.e. with clinical improvement in hours or days, and it may be visible only when the patient looks in the direction of the nystagmus fast phase. Nystagmus in all three horizontal positions of gaze is called *third-degree nystagmus*; nystagmus with gaze straight ahead and in the direction of the fast phase is called *second-degree nystagmus*; whereas nystagmus appearing only while looking in the direction of the fast phase is called *first-degree nystagmus*.

Video 03.01 – Left-sided vestibular neuritis
This patient developed acute vertigo five days earlier and was considerably improved when the video was taken. There is a minimal degree of right-beating nystagmus in primary gaze; this enhances on gaze deviation to the right and is abolished on left gaze. The nystagmus becomes clearly visible when Frenzel's glasses are worn, i.e. when optic fixation is removed. The final section of this video clip shows further enhancement of the right-beating nystagmus after head shaking.

symptoms. A way of solving this dilemma is to think that both the eyes and the body tend to drift towards the lesion side, and then corrective movements, such as the fast phases of nystagmus develop. Further confirmation of the suspected side will come from finding an abnormal (positive) head-impulse test when rotating the head towards the lesion.

- *A positive head-impulse test.* Unilateral vestibular failure can be demonstrated by rapidly turning the patient's head to either side (see page 36; video clip 03.02). With acute vestibular neuritis on the right, the vestibulo-ocular reflex is defective when the nose is turned to the right. Thus, visual fixation cannot be maintained during the head rotation and, instead, the eyes move with the head (see Figure 2.2). It takes the patient only half a second to realise that he or she is off target and to make a quick corrective eye movement for refixation (see video clips 02.13 and 3.02). The corrective eye movement can be easily distinguished from the spontaneous nystagmus beats as it is considerably bigger, provided that head rotations are fast and sufficiently large (around 20 degrees).

- *Veering towards the affected ear.* This is either obvious from observing the patient while he/she walks around or can be formally tested with the Romberg test (see Chapter 2). After eye closure or when standing heel-to-toe (tandem-Romberg position) directional imbalance becomes even more evident.

Video 03.02 – Abnormal head-thrust test to the left
Patient shown in video clip 03.01 – Left-sided vestibular neuritis. Note small corrective 'catch-up' saccades during left head turns.

Pathophysiology

Viral infection is the most probable cause of vestibular neuritis. Arguments supporting this hypothesis include (mini-)epidemics of vestibular neuritis, the frequent association with viral infections, demonstration of latent herpes simplex virus type 1 in human vestibular ganglia, and a few postmortem studies which showed post-inflammatory changes on the vestibular nerve. An ischaemic component may be superimposed when swelling of the nerve within its bony canal compromises blood flow.

The clinical signs and symptoms of vestibular neuritis can be logically inferred from vestibular physiology. Remember that even when the head is upright and at rest there is a constant flow of afferent signals from the semicircular canals and otoliths. Movements or positional changes of the head activate one labyrinth and inhibit the other, which leads to an increased input from one side and a decreased input from the other. The resulting asymmetry of neuronal activity in the vestibular nuclei produces compensatory eye movements and postural adjustments, and makes us sense our head movement and position. When the input from one side comes to a halt due to vestibular neuritis, neuronal activity in the ipsilateral vestibular nucleus will stop while the contralateral nucleus is still active. The resulting asymmetrical firing corresponds to an apparent continuous head rotation to the healthy side. Thus the resting activity in the vestibulo-ocular reflex is also biased and generates drifting eye movements opposing the apparent head rotation; i.e. toward the affected side. These are interrupted by resetting fast phases in the opposite direction, producing the net result of a spontaneous nystagmus beating to the healthy side (Figure 3.2). Similarly, vertical canal and otolith involvement are responsible for the small torsional component of the nystagmus and for the tilt sensation and lateropulsion leading to ipsilesional falls.

Investigations

Vestibular neuritis is a clinical diagnosis. Therefore, when a patient matches the above criteria and has no other neurological signs, no further testing is required. Video-oculography with caloric testing or the video head-impulse test are often employed to document the unilateral loss of vestibular function and to monitor recovery. Audiometry can be useful to document associated sensorineural hearing loss which would point to an alternative diagnosis such as labyrinthine infarction (see page 67), Ménière's disease (see page 79) or perilymph fistula (see page 88). Magnetic resonance imaging (MRI) is required only when neurological symptoms indicate brainstem or cerebellar involvement or when a sudden onset of symptoms in a patient with vascular risk factors suggests an ischaemic event. Inflammation of the nerve itself is usually not visible on MRI. Computed tomography (CT) is not a suitable alternative as it notoriously fails to visualise small brainstem and cerebellar lesions. Searching for a virus is unrewarding and cannot prove a causal relationship at the current state of knowledge.

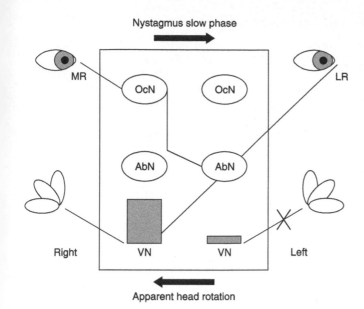

Nystagmus slow phase

MR

OcN   OcN   LR

AbN   AbN

Right   VN   VN   Left

Apparent head rotation

Figure 3.2 Brainstem mechanism generating spontaneous nystagmus due to vestibular neuritis on the left. Level of neuronal activity within the vestibular nuclei is indicated by vertical bars. Asymmetries between the vestibular nuclei lead to asymmetric activation of the vestibulo-ocular reflex arc which generates slow eye movements opposing the perceived head rotation (slow phases of nystagmus). The fast phase of nystagmus beats in the opposite direction, i.e. to the healthy ear. VN = vestibular nuclei, AbN = abducens nuclei, OcN = oculomotor nuclei, MR = medial rectus muscle, LR = lateral rectus muscle.

Differential diagnosis

Cranial-nerve, brainstem and cerebellar function as well as hearing should be specifically examined in all patients presenting with persistent vertigo. When clinical findings are not consistent with vestibular neuritis, immediate referral to neurology (or to ENT for suspected inner-ear disease) is mandatory. The worst case scenario would be missing a cerebellar infarct or haemorrhage, with subsequent hydrocephalus leading to brainstem herniation. 'Red flags' for acute central vestibular lesions, typically posterior fossa stroke, are listed in Table 3.3.

Central lesions, particularly strokes causing vertigo, can be differentiated from vestibular neuritis on the basis of clinical examination:

- a normal head-impulse test indicating normal peripheral function (one of the few exceptions in medicine when a *negative* finding, i.e. a *normal* head-impulse test, indicates a more sinister underlying diagnosis);
- a nystagmus which changes direction depending on direction of gaze, or any other central-looking nystagmus such as up- or downbeat nystagmus;
- skew deviation, i.e. a vertical misalignment of the eyes, which is best detected by covering either eye in an alternating fashion. When uncovered, the upper eye will move downwards for fixation and vice versa (see video clips 03.03 and 03.04).

When one of these three signs is present, a central lesion is highly likely. This approach has been summarised by the acronym HINTS, which stands for: **H**ead Impulse, **N**ystagmus, and **T**esting for **S**kew. When properly applied, it can be more sensitive than MRI at initial presentation. Further signs for a central lesion include:

- prominent ataxia which often makes patients unable to stand on their own whereas patients with vestibular neuritis can usually stand as long as they keep their eyes open;
- other cerebellar and brainstem signs such as broken-up pursuit, asymmetric saccades, defective suppression of the vestibulo-ocular reflex, limb ataxia, dysarthria, swallowing difficulty, weakness or sensory loss;

Table 3.3 Acute vertigo: pointers to posterior circulation stroke

Negative (= normal) head-impulse test

Nystagmus in more than one direction

Ocular skew deviation or any central ocular–motor abnormality

Hemianopia

Severe occipital headache

Unilateral deafness

Severe truncal ataxia or inability to stand or walk

Any brainstem or cerebellar sign

Video 03.03 – Small skew deviation
The alternating cover test is useful to detect a small degree of vertical misalignment of the eyes (skew deviation). The patient is asked to fixate the examiner's nose. You will note that that the upper (hypertropic eye) moves downward when uncovered while the lower (hypotropic) eye moves upward for fixation.

Video 03.04 – Large skew deviation
A large skew deviation is visible at first sight as in this patient with Wernicke's encephalopathy. Note that the angle of vertical squint remains constant in all directions of gaze. A separate finding in this patient is bilateral gaze-evoked nystagmus.

- normal cold-water calorics (20 °C) applied at the bedside using a 20–50 ml syringe which produces a horizontal nystagmus to the opposite ear. (In contrast, patients with vestibular neuritis show an unaltered spontaneous nystagmus when syringed on the affected side and attenuation of the spontaneous nystagmus when the healthy ear is irrigated.)

For a synoptic differential diagnosis of acute vertigo with spontaneous nystagmus, see Table 3.6 (on page 63). More details on these disorders are presented in the following sections of this chapter.

Natural course

The approach to treatment of vestibular neuritis can be summarised by three key messages:

1. All patients improve spontaneously and few have residual symptoms.
2. Vestibular exercises accelerate recovery by promoting central compensation.
3. Long-term morbidity depends more on psychological than physical factors.

Peripheral vestibular function is restored in about half of the patients within a couple of months. Clinical recovery, however, usually progresses at a faster pace and is mostly unrelated to intact peripheral function: most patients become mobile within a week or two and largely symptom-free after two or three months. Minor residual symptoms include brief oscillopsia and imbalance during rapid head turns towards the affected side. Fewer than 20% of patients retain bothersome symptoms such as chronic disequilibrium, head-motion intolerance and often anxiety with avoidance behaviour. Many of these patients have anxious personality traits and experience high levels of anxiety during the acute stage of vestibular loss. This may lead to catastrophic thoughts, enhanced vigilance of vestibular signals and a cautious way of controlling balance and moving around. All these maladaptive strategies tend to persist even after acute symptoms have ceased. It is crucial to identify patients at risk as early as possible to prevent chronic morbidity by counselling, encouraging physical activity and customised vestibular rehabilitation. Other risk factors for incomplete recovery include old age, underlying CNS disease and enhanced visual dependence (see visual vertigo, Chapter 6).

Benign paroxysmal positional vertigo (BPPV) involving the posterior canal on the affected side develops in about 20–30% of patients and can be treated by repositioning manoeuvres (see page 108). BPPV as a complication of vestibular neuritis appears paradoxical at first sight, as a dead labyrinth should not produce any excitatory symptoms. Several studies, however, have shown that the inferior division of the vestibular nerve supplying the posterior semicircular canal is usually spared in vestibular neuritis. Thus, the posterior canal can be activated by mobile otoconia which have dissolved from the damaged utricular macula (see page 108).

Patients with a previous history of vestibular neuritis will be completely normal on clinical examination, when peripheral function has fully recovered. With persistent peripheral failure, routine tests are also normal, but several simple procedures will help to unmask the deficit:

- *Frenzel's glasses* may show a subtle residual spontaneous nystagmus towards the healthy side.
- *Ophthalmoscopy* with the other eye covered is even more sensitive for detection of spontaneous nystagmus, but remember that nystagmus direction is reversed on the back of the eye.
- *Head-shaking*, performed vigorously for 20 seconds, temporarily increases asymmetrical activity in the vestibular nuclei, thus producing nystagmus for a few seconds towards the healthy ear. Head-shaking nystagmus is best observed with Frenzel's glasses.
- *Head-impulse testing* can remain abnormal for a lifetime in patients with unilateral loss of at least 50%.
- The 'sharpened' or *tandem-Romberg*, the Unterberger test or walking with eyes closed can all identify a tendency to veer or fall towards the damaged side, but perform the test at least three times to check for reproducibility! (See examination in Chapter 2.)

The process that leads to cessation of vertigo and spontaneous nystagmus after unilateral vestibular loss is called *central compensation*. The essential mechanism for central compensation is restoration of spontaneous activity in the vestibular nucleus on the affected side, which is deprived of peripheral input. Once symmetrical firing of central vestibular neurons is achieved, spontaneous nystagmus disappears. In addition, neuronal activity on the affected side can be modulated by peripheral input from the intact side which is transmitted by an inhibitory pathway across the midline. This enhances the vestibulo-ocular reflex for head turns towards the affected side, at least in the low- and medium-velocity range (Figure 3.3).

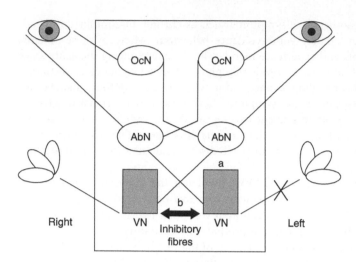

Figure 3.3 Central compensation of a unilateral peripheral vestibular lesion. a: Restoration of neuronal activity in the vestibular nucleus on the affected side in the absence of peripheral input, leading to cessation of spontaneous nystagmus (static compensation). b: Modulation of neuronal activity in the deafferented vestibular nucleus from the intact side via inhibitory brainstem pathways crossing the midline (dynamic compensation).

Treatment

Treatment of the acute phase includes a short period of bed-rest and vestibular suppressants (e.g. 150 mg dimenhydrinate suppositories twice a day). This should be discontinued after two days because, at least in experimental animals, sedating substances retard vestibular compensation. At this stage patients are usually able to begin vestibular exercises which have been shown to accelerate recovery of postural balance (Figure 3.4). Vestibular exercises include visual and postural tasks as well as complex movements which stimulate multisensory integration and eye–head coordination. Details of vestibular rehabilitation can be found in Chapter 8. A typical patient can leave hospital within a week with an instruction for continued exercises at home for another four to eight weeks. As many patients with acute vestibular neuritis are not hospitalised, it is essential to explain to the patient and family that early mobilisation (even if it causes dizziness) is essential for recovery.

The role for steroids as a treatment for acute vestibular neuritis is debated. A randomised trial indicated that an initial dose of 100 mg methylprednisolone slowly tapered over three weeks increased the rate of peripheral recovery from 40 to 60% (caloric tests). However, a separate trial showed no improvement in long-term clinical outcome, in agreement with the fact that laboratory vestibular tests do not predict outcome.

Brainstem and cerebellar lesions

Fortunately, brainstem and cerebellar lesions are uncommon causes of acute vertigo, accounting for fewer than 20% of vertiginous patients presenting to an emergency department. On the other hand, in patients above 60 with one or more vascular risk factors, the proportion rises to over 50%. One would not like to miss a single such patient because of the grave consequences, which can be avoided by appropriate management. An example is thrombolysis in a patient with incipient basilar artery thrombosis. CT imaging of all patients presenting with acute vertigo is not an easy way out of this dilemma because it is neither cost-effective nor sufficiently sensitive and specific. Early ischaemia and small areas of demyelination may be invisible and, all too often, an incidental brainstem or cerebellar lesion unrelated to central vestibular

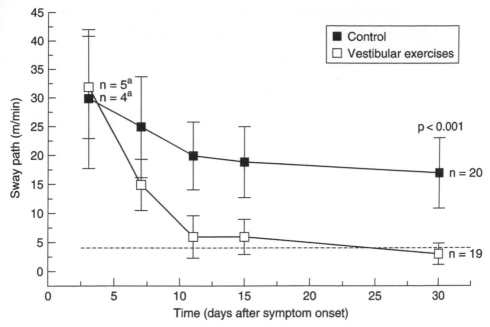

Figure 3.4 Imbalance in patients with vestibular neuritis treated with vestibular exercises and in untreated controls. Imbalance is expressed as a sway path (m/min) measured on a posturographic platform. Exercises were applied three times daily for 30 minutes over 30 days. The dotted line indicates the upper limit of the normal range. (From: Strupp, Arbusov et al., with permission.)

structures will be blamed for the patient's symptoms. Therefore, clinical criteria must be applied to select patients for brain MRI to increase the probability of identifying a relevant lesion (Table 3.4).

Disorders of the brainstem and cerebellum can be classified according to anatomy or aetiology. Anatomical localisation is usually possible on the basis of clinical findings while aetiology is reflected by the temporal evolution of symptoms (Table 3.5). In the following, disorders will be discussed as localisation-related syndromes. A specific, namely vascular, aetiology can be implied when clinical signs are related to an arterial territory. Conversely, non-vascular lesions (e.g. demyelinating) do not respect vascular territories and produce individual deficits relating to size and anatomical involvement.

Table 3.6 provides an overview of the posterior fossa and inner-ear syndromes presenting with acute vertigo with special regard to nystagmus patterns and associated findings.

Brainstem lesion at the root entry zone of the vestibular nerve

Rarely, a small area of infarction or demyelination at the root entry zone of the vestibular nerve may mimic vestibular neuritis, interrupting the flow of peripheral vestibular input into the vestibular nuclei at brainstem level. This is sometimes called *pseudo*-vestibular neuritis. Apart from the usual symptoms and signs of vestibular neuritis there are additional features that should raise the suspicion of a root entry lesion: abrupt or hyper-acute onset with a background of vascular risk factors (ischaemia?); previous episodes of unexplained neurological dysfunction (MS?); and associated findings resulting from involvement of adjacent structures, such as distorted hearing (cochlear nerve and nucleus),

Table 3.4 Clinical criteria for requesting magnetic resonance imaging in a patient with acute vertigo

Clinical criterion	Suspected diagnosis
Abrupt onset of vertigo against a background of old age or vascular risk factors	Ischaemia of the labyrinth or root entry zone of the eighth nerve?
Abrupt onset of profound hearing loss	Labyrinthine infarction (i.e. due to AICA occlusion)? Concomitant brainstem/cerebellar infarction?
Previous episodes of unexplained neurological symptoms for days or weeks in a young patient	Undiagnosed MS, acute lesion in the root entry zone of the eighth nerve?
Spontaneous nystagmus with *normal* head-impulse test	Central vestibular or cerebellar lesion?
Central oculomotor findings: nystagmus in more than one direction, skew deviation[a] saccadic pursuit, pure torsional nystagmus, upbeat/downbeat nystagmus, central positional nystagmus	Involvement of central vestibular structures in the brainstem or cerebellum?
Cranial nerve abnormalities	Brainstem lesion or tumour/inflammation close to the brainstem?
Long tract signs: hemi-/quadriparesis, extensor plantar responses, hemisensory loss, Horner's syndrome	Brainstem lesion?
Cerebellar signs: truncal/limb ataxia, dysarthria	Cerebellar lesion?

[a] Skew deviation designates a vertical misalignment of the eyes of central origin. In contrast to squints resulting from paresis of extra-ocular muscles, skew deviations show a stable squint in all directions of gaze (see video clips 03.03 and 03.04).
AICA = anterior inferior cerebellar artery; MS = multiple sclerosis

Table 3.5 Progression and course of brainstem/cerebellar syndromes as a clue to aetiology

Temporal course	Likely aetiology
Abrupt onset, duration: few minutes to two hours (rarely longer)	Transient ischaemic attack
Abrupt onset, duration: days to permanent	Stroke
Progression over days, resolution over days to weeks	Inflammation, demyelination
Progression over days to weeks	Carcinomatous meningitis, paraneoplastic disease, malignant tumour, metastasis
Progression over weeks to months	Malignant tumour, metastasis
Progression over years	Benign tumour (e.g. meningioma), low-grade glioma, degenerative disorder

Table 3.6 Nystagmus features and associated findings in disorders presenting with acute prolonged vertigo

Disorder/ syndrome	Nystagmus features	Associated findings
Vestibular neuritis	Horizontal–torsional towards healthy side	Veering towards lesioned side, abnormal head-impulse test
Labyrinthine infarction	Horizontal–torsional towards healthy side	Veering towards lesioned side, abnormal head-impulse test, hearing loss
Herpes Zoster oticus	Horizontal–torsional towards healthy side	Veering towards lesioned side, abnormal head-impulse test, hearing loss, facial palsy, vesicles in the external auditory canal
Brainstem lesion at the root entry of the vestibular nerve	Horizontal–torsional towards healthy side	Possible: decreased/distorted hearing, skew deviation, abnormal pursuit, hemiataxia, Horner's syndrome
Isolated lesion of one vestibular nucleus	Pure torsional towards healthy side (frequent) or any other (rare)	Ocular tilt reaction, saccadic pursuit
Complete infarction of the AICA	Horizontal–torsional towards healthy side (vestibular nystagmus) and gaze-evoked nystagmus towards lesioned side (cerebellar nystagmus)	*Ipsilesional*: signs of unilateral vestibular loss, profound hearing loss, Horner's syndrome, loss of sensation on the face, facial paralysis, limb and truncal ataxia *Contralesional*: loss of sensation on the body
Complete infarction of the PICA	Often horizontal–torsional towards healthy side (vestibular nystagmus) and gaze-evoked nystagmus towards lesioned side (cerebellar nystagmus)	*Ipsilesional*: facial paralysis, vocal cord paralysis, palatal paresis, decreased gag reflex, Horner's syndrome, loss of temperature and pain sensation on the face, limb and trunk ataxia *Contralesional*: ocular tilt reaction, loss of temperature and pain sensation on the body
Isolated hemispheric cerebellar lesion	Ipsilateral gaze-evoked nystagmus	*Ipsilesional*: saccadic pursuit, defective VOR suppression, limb ataxia *and*: truncal ataxia, dysarthria
Bilateral lesion of cerebellar flocculus	Bilateral gaze-evoked nystagmus	*Bilateral*: saccadic pursuit, defective VOR suppression, truncal ataxia
Acute Ménière attack	Horizontal–torsional towards affected or healthy side	Unilateral tinnitus, hearing loss, aural fullness/pressure
Acute attack of vestibular migraine	Any type of spontaneous or persistent positional nystagmus	Unsteadiness (common), other posterior fossa symptoms (rare)

AICA/PICA = anterior/posterior inferior cerebellar artery; VOR = vestibulo-ocular reflex

Video 03.05 – Pure torsional nystagmus
The video clip shows a patient in the upright position with a torsional nystagmus beating towards the left ear. The nystagmus is continually beating towards the left. Pure torsional spontaneous nystagmus indicates a lesion of the contralateral vestibular nucleus. The influence of positioning on this central nystagmus is shown in video clip 05.14 – Atypical (central) positional nystagmus.

Horner's syndrome (sympathetic pathway in the lateral brainstem), facial paralysis (facial-nerve root entry zone), saccadic (broken-up) pursuit eye movements (cerebellum), and ipsilateral limb ataxia (cerebellar peduncle and cerebellum). Magnetic resonance imaging will usually visualise the lesion.

Isolated lesion of one vestibular nucleus

Most lesions of the vestibular nuclei occur in conjunction with infarction of the anterior or posterior inferior cerebellar artery territories. Occasionally, however, a vascular or demyelinating lesion may be restricted to the vestibular nucleus or, more precisely, to one or several of the four vestibular subnuclei on one side. The resulting clinical findings vary with the subnuclei involved, but a purely torsional or mixed torsional–horizontal nystagmus towards the healthy ear with a moderate caloric paresis on the affected side seems to be the most common pattern (video clip 03.05). As the final path of smooth-pursuit eye movements travels from the cerebellum through the vestibular nuclei to the ocular motor neurons, impairment of smooth pursuit is commonly associated. An ocular tilt reaction (skew deviation with the ipsilateral eye down, ipsiversive ocular torsion and head tilt) may result from involvement of the upper half of the vestibular nucleus.

Complete infarction of the anterior inferior cerebellar artery (AICA) territory

The AICA supplies three arterial territories all of which are part of the vestibular system:
- the labyrinth (cochlear and vestibular) and eighth nerve;
- the lateral brainstem at pontine level including the root entry zone of the eighth nerve and part of the vestibular nuclei;
- a variable portion of the lateral cerebellum including the cerebellar peduncles and the flocculus.

Therefore, complete infarction of the AICA territory produces a variety of symptoms, including a mixed peripheral and central pattern of vestibular dysfunction:
- Horizontal–torsional spontaneous nystagmus to the healthy side, an abnormal head-thrust test and hearing loss (labyrinth and eighth nerve). Selective loss of hearing or vestibular function is rare.
- Horner's syndrome, facial paralysis and sensory loss, and crossed hemisensory loss to pain and temperature on the body (lateral pons). Variable involvement of parts of the vestibular nucleus may modify the labyrinthine spontaneous nystagmus.
- Gait ataxia, ipsilateral limb dysmetria, asymmetrically impaired smooth pursuit, and bilateral gaze-evoked nystagmus (cerebellum).

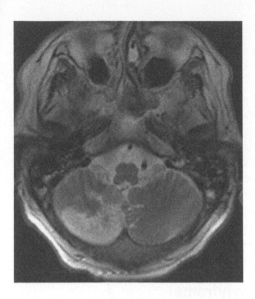

Figure 3.5 Cerebellar stroke. Magnetic resonance image showing selective infarction of the cerebellar branch of the right posterior inferior cerebellar artery with sparing of the lateral medulla.

Branch occlusion may lead to partial infarction of the AICA territory with limited clinical symptoms only. On the other hand, bilateral symptoms from the AICA territory can be an early manifestation of basilar artery thrombosis. When large portions of the cerebellum are supplied by the AICA, extended infarcts may develop with cerebellar swelling and subsequent brainstem herniation. Therefore, rapid imaging is critical. Follow-up studies have shown that hearing and peripheral vestibular function improve in most patients after labyrinthine ischaemia.

Complete infarction of the posterior inferior cerebellar artery (PICA) territory (Wallenberg's syndrome)

The PICA supplies the lateral medulla including the vestibular nuclei and most of the caudal cerebellum. Infarction of the PICA territory, usually caused by dissection or occlusion of the vertebral artery, causes diverse nystagmus patterns, most commonly a horizontal–torsional spontaneous nystagmus beating towards the intact side and gaze-evoked nystagmus towards the affected side. Ipsilesional and alternating spontaneous nystagmus may also occur. A skew deviation with the ipsilateral eye deviated downward occurs in about half of the patients; some have an associated ipsilesional head tilt (so-called *ocular tilt reaction*). Associated ipsilesional findings include falls to the affected side, saccadic pursuit, limb ataxia, trigeminal sensory loss to pain and temperature, facial paralysis, decreased gag reflex, hoarseness due to vocal cord paralysis, dysphagia, Horner's syndrome, decreased sweating, and (on the contralesional side) hemisensory loss to pain and temperature. Incomplete Wallenberg's syndromes are common due to individual variations of the vascular territory and isolated occlusion of the brainstem or cerebellar branches (Figure 3.5). The main difference from AICA infarction is preservation of hearing and involvement of lower cranial nerves.

Isolated cerebellar lesion

An isolated cerebellar lesion causes vertigo only when it involves caudal cerebellar structures which interact with the vestibular nuclei such as the flocculus, nodulus, uvula and some deep cerebellar nuclei. Lesions of the cerebellar vermis result in unsteadiness and truncal ataxia but not in vertigo. In cerebellar disease the nystagmus is usually gaze-evoked, rather than spontaneous, and has a larger amplitude. However, a unilateral lesion of the caudal cerebellum due to partial PICA infarction may cause spontaneous horizontal nystagmus to the affected side by disinhibiting the ipsilateral vestibular nucleus. In fact, this is the most common mimic of vestibular neuritis. A normal head-impulse test, normal caloric responses, and gaze-evoked nystagmus when the patient looks in the opposite direction of his spontaneous nystagmus, will point to the correct diagnosis. Isolated lesions of the nodulus may present with ipsilesional spontaneous nystagmus or periodic alternating nystagmus, which is a spontaneous nystagmus that changes direction every one or two minutes.

A subacute bilateral cerebellar syndrome usually indicates drug toxicity (see page 105) and less commonly cerebellitis or paraneoplastic cerebellar degeneration.

Herpes zoster oticus (Ramsay Hunt syndrome)

When acute unilateral vestibulopathy is associated with a painful ear and facial paralysis you should suspect herpes zoster oticus. Hearing loss and tinnitus is often associated. Vesicles in the external ear canal or on the auricle confirm the diagnosis. Meningitis, encephalitis, cranial polyneuropathy or cerebellar involvement occur less frequently. Most patients have a prodromal phase with ear and head pain for a few days. Herpes zoster ('shingles') is caused by reactivation of the varicella zoster virus, which causes chickenpox in children and persists in sensory ganglia. Cranial MRI typically shows increased signal of inner-ear soft tissues on FLAIR images. Early treatment with aciclovir (30 mg/kg per day in three divided doses for one or two weeks) is advised, particularly in immunocompromised patients. Aciclovir may also help to prevent postherpetic neuralgia. The acute peripheral vestibular loss is treated with a vestibular suppressant for one to three days and vestibular rehabilitation exercises.

First attack of vestibular migraine

One of the first questions to ask a patient with acute vertigo is whether he or she has had this before. When the answer is 'yes', the differential diagnosis narrows down to the disorders discussed in Chapter 4, with vestibular migraine, Ménière's disease and transient ischaemic attacks (TIAs) ranging at the top of the list. But even if the answer is 'no', it is worthwhile to enquire about similar attacks of lesser intensity which may lead to a correct diagnosis. When one is actually dealing with a first-ever attack, it is still possible that it is the first manifestation of a recurrent disorder. Vestibular migraine is a relevant differential diagnosis in this situation as it is common and can present with all types of central and peripheral spontaneous nystagmus as well as central positional nystagmus. Associated ataxia or other central findings may mimic a vertebrobasilar stroke. The diagnosis is supported by a history of migraine and migraine features during the attack, such as headaches, photophobia, phonophobia or aura symptoms. However, the diagnosis can be confirmed only when similar attacks have recurred several times. Therefore, magnetic resonance imaging is advisable when a patient presents with a first attack of suspected vestibular migraine and ongoing symptoms. For further details on vestibular migraine, see page 71.

First attack of BPPV

Although BPPV is by definition a cause of recurrent vertigo, the first episode is a traumatic experience for most patients, and large numbers of patients with BPPV are seen for their first attack in emergency rooms. Both on retrospective interrogation and during the acute emergency admission, doctors are frequently misled by patients interpreting their symptoms as due to a single, long-duration attack of continuous vertigo. This is probably the result of the patients not being able to identify which specific movements of the head trigger the episodes – as far as they are concerned anything they do brings on vertigo. Most patients believe that they are experiencing a heart attack or a stroke. Details of the various forms of BPPV and their treatment are extensively discussed in Chapter 5. Here it suffices to say that any patient with a first attack of vertigo who does not have a clear vestibular neuritis (unidirectional horizontal nystagmus and a positive head-impulse test) or a posterior fossa stroke (positive neurological symptoms or findings) should undergo posterior canal and horizontal canal diagnostic manoeuvres.

First attack of Ménière's disease

With a usual duration between 20 minutes and several hours, Ménière attacks have often abated once patients are seen in an emergency room. On examination, one may observe either the secondary inhibitory nystagmus beating towards the healthy ear, or the tertiary recovery nystagmus beating towards the affected ear. In a patient with a first manifestation of Ménière's disease the diagnosis is facilitated when there is concomitant hearing loss, tinnitus and aural fullness. However, Ménière's disease often starts monosymptomatically with either isolated cochlear symptoms (more common) or vestibular symptoms (less common). Therefore, a previous history of fluctuating hearing loss and tinnitus can provide valuable information whereas a first episode of isolated vertigo may be difficult to interpret. Careful follow-up including audiometry is advisable, since most patients with Ménière's disease will experience the full spectrum of symptoms within a year or two. When vertigo recurs and cochlear symptoms are still missing after one year, a diagnosis of vestibular migraine is much more likely. For further details of Ménière's disease, see page 79.

Other causes of acute persistent vertigo

Labyrinthine infarction may result from selective occlusion of the labyrinthine artery, which usually originates from the anterior inferior cerebellar artery and sometimes directly from the basilar artery. As the labyrinthine artery irrigates both the cochlea and the vestibular labyrinth, simultaneous hearing loss and vertigo is to be expected. The typical presentation would be an elderly patient with vascular risk factors, abrupt onset of symptoms and possibly preceding brief episodes of vertigo implying labyrinthine TIAs.

Perilymph fistula can likewise present with prolonged vertigo with or without hearing symptoms. The diagnosis is doubtful, however, in the absence of an inciting event such as ear surgery, direct trauma or sudden pressure changes, or a history of cholesteatoma. For further details of perilymph fistula, see page 88.

Bacterial labyrinthitis has become rare in the antibiotic era. It may occur as a complication of otitis media or mastoiditis, either with direct bacterial invasion (suppurative labyrinthitis) or with spread of bacterial toxins into the inner ear (serous labyrinthitis).

Unilateral sensorineural hearing loss and vertigo occur with both variants but are much more pronounced with suppurative labyrinthitis. Treatment includes antibiotics and surgical eradication of the middle ear and mastoid infection.

Another route for bacteria to invade the labyrinth is through the cerebrospinal fluid (CSF). Therefore, patients with bacterial meningitis may develop bilateral labyrinthitis, often leading to permanent hearing and vestibular loss. Antibiotics are the mainstay of treatment for bacterial labyrinthitis and surgery is indicated only when there is a chronic ear infection or epidural abscess.

Drug or alcohol toxicity will be all too familiar to any emergency room doctor, so only a few points have to be stressed here. When dizziness (rather than vertigo) and imbalance are the key symptoms, cerebellar toxicity is the most likely mechanism. Examination shows gaze-evoked nystagmus, saccadic pursuit, dysarthria, gait ataxia and, usually less pronounced, limb ataxia. The offending drugs include antiepileptics such as phenytoin, carbamazepine and lamotrigine, as well as lithium and benzodiazepines. Alcohol intoxication presents in a similar way but often with the addition of nystagmus in both lateral head positions (so-called positional alcohol nystagmus). This nystagmus results from alcohol penetrating the labyrinth and beats to the lower ear in the early phase of intoxication (hours 1–3) and to the upper ear in the late phase (hours 5–10).

What to do if you don't have a clue

When a patient presents during an episode of acute vertigo a diagnosis can usually be made on the basis of the clinical examination (see Table 3.6, page 63).

Is the physical examination entirely normal?

If it is, the commonest reasons are these:

- *The attack is just over.* The patient should confirm that the vertigo is gone, while he or she may continue to feel nauseated for a while. Then, a diagnosis has to be based on the patient's history and results from vestibular testing and audiometry. Imaging is rarely helpful in this situation because short-lived attacks are usually not related to a structural lesion.
- *The disorder does not involve prominent findings during attacks.* Some patients with vestibular migraine have a seasick type of vertigo and feel very ill, but present with just some mild imbalance on Romberg testing and no spontaneous nystagmus. Enquire about additional migraine features.
- *The patient has non-vestibular dizziness rather than vertigo.* In the emergency room setting, common causes of dizziness include: hypertensive crises, hypoglycaemia or other metabolic problems, and panic attacks with or without hyperventilation.

Are there signs suggesting brainstem or cerebellar disease, but imaging is negative?

When confronted with a vertiginous patient with clear-cut central signs such as upbeat or downbeat nystagmus, gaze-evoked nystagmus, saccadic pursuit or ataxia, but with normal magnetic resonance imaging, you should consider the following disorders:

- *Negative on imaging*

- – vestibular migraine
- – TIA/early stroke (may show unrelated vascular lesions)
- – drug toxicity, particularly due to antiepileptics or lithium
- – paraneoplastic subacute cerebellar degeneration (negative imaging during the first few months)

- *Sometimes negative on imaging*
  - – very small brainstem stroke
  - – brainstem encephalitis (viral, autoimmune)
  - – cerebellitis (viral, autoimmune).

Multiple sclerosis is another possibility in this context because small demyelinating lesions within the brainstem often cannot be visualised, but usually there are periventricular lesions pointing to that diagnosis.

Chapter 4

Recurrent vertigo and dizziness

This chapter focuses on recurrent attacks of vertigo or dizziness. The two symptoms are discussed separately because they can often be distinguished by their clinical presentation. In clinical practice, this distinction can help to limit the number of differential diagnoses that have to be considered.

- *Vertigo* involves a spinning sensation or other types of illusory motion of the self or the environment. The visual illusion of a rotating environment is particularly useful and should be specifically enquired about. Vertigo is often accompanied by nausea, vomiting and imbalance and is often aggravated by head movements and changes of head position. This combination of symptoms implies acute dysfunction in peripheral or central vestibular structures – in this chapter as a recurrent form.
- *Dizziness* is a less specific symptom. It may comprise sensations such as light-headedness, wooziness, giddiness, impending faint and sometimes even tiredness, difficulty in concentrating and anxiety (see page 93).

There are exceptions from this dichotomy, such as occasional patients with panic attacks or orthostatic hypotension, who report vertigo rather than dizziness. Conversely, mild vestibular dysfunction may present with dizziness rather than vertigo. However, the disorders from the *vertigo* section below usually cause unequivocal vestibular symptoms at some stage of the disease and not dizziness alone.

Most patients with recurrent vertigo or dizziness are seen during the asymptomatic interval, which makes the physical examination often unrewarding. Thus, careful history-taking is critical for accurate diagnosis. Type of dizziness, duration of attacks, accompanying symptoms and precipitating factors need to be explored.

Recurrent *positional* vertigo is discussed separately in Chapter 5.

RECURRENT VERTIGO

Table 4.1 Recurrent vertigo: diagnoses with key features (for recurrent dizziness see page 93)

Disorder	Key features
Vestibular migraine (page 71)	Attacks of spontaneous or positional vertigo lasting minutes to days; history of migraine; migraine symptoms during vertigo; migraine-specific precipitants provoking vertigo
Probable vestibular migraine (page 73)	Same clinical features as vestibular migraine, but relationship to migraine is less obvious, e.g. no personal history of migraine or lack of migraine symptoms during the attack

Table 4.1 (*cont.*)

Disorder	Key features
Ménière's disease (page 79)	Vertigo attacks lasting 20 minutes to several hours with concurrent hearing loss, tinnitus and aural fullness Progressive hearing loss over years
Vertebrobasilar TIA (page 84)	Attacks of vertigo lasting minutes, often accompanied by ataxia, dysarthria, diplopia or visual-field defects Affects older adults with vascular risk factors
Vestibular paroxysmia (page 86)	Brief attacks of vertigo (seconds) several times per day with or without cochlear symptoms; often good response to carbamazepine Often caused by vascular compression of the eighth nerve
Benign paroxysmal positional vertigo (BPPV) (page 108)	BPPV and other recurrent vertigo that is *provoked by changes of head position* is dealt with separately in Chapter 5
Other rare causes (page 89)	Perilymph fistula, superior canal dehiscence, autoimmune inner-ear disease, syphilis of the inner ear, schwannoma of the eighth nerve, vestibular epilepsy, insufficient compensation of unilateral vestibular loss, otosclerosis, Paget's disease, episodic ataxia type 2, familial hemiplegic migraine

Vestibular migraine

Table 4.2 Vestibular migraine: key features

History	Attacks of variable duration with spontaneous vertigo, positional vertigo, head motion-induced dizziness or visually induced dizziness, accompanied by one or several migraine symptoms such as headache, photophobia, phonophobia or auras Sometimes migraine-specific precipitants such as hormonal changes or lack of sleep
Clinical findings	During the asymptomatic interval: usually normal During attacks: central or peripheral spontaneous nystagmus, central positional nystagmus, ataxia
Pathophysiology	Unknown. Ion-channel dysfunction? Imbalance of neurotransmitters? Spreading depression?
Investigations	A first acute episode may require imaging to rule out posterior fossa lesion Video-oculography, caloric testing and audiometry may be abnormal – not frequently and findings are non-specific
Treatment	Vestibular suppressants or triptans for acute attacks, migraine prophylaxis for frequent and severe attacks Sufficient evidence from controlled studies is lacking

Clinical features

Vestibular migraine is the most common cause of recurrent spontaneous vertigo and the second most common vestibular disorder after benign paroxysmal positional vertigo. It affects 10 to 20% of all migraine patients and accounts for about 10% of referrals to specialised dizziness clinics. Vestibular migraine may start at any age and has a female preponderance of about 3:1. Familial occurrence is not rare, pointing to a genetic origin of the disorder. In 2013, vestibular migraine was recognised by the International Classification of Headache Disorders (ICHD-III). Previous terms for this condition were migrainous vertigo, migraine-related dizziness, migraine-associated vertigo, and any combination of these names.

The term *migraine with brainstem aura* (formerly called 'basilar migraine') should be restricted to patients who fulfil the respective ICHD-III criteria, including at least two aura symptoms from the brainstem such as dysarthria, vertigo, tinnitus, hearing loss, ataxia, diplopia or decreased level of consciousness and a duration of 5–60 minutes for each aura symptom. In addition, patients should have at least one of the more usual migraine aura symptoms (visual, sensory, language-related) during the same attack. In fact, fewer than 5% of patients with vestibular migraine correspond to this pattern. *Benign paroxysmal vertigo of childhood* designates a variant of vestibular migraine that starts at pre-school age with brief attacks of isolated vertigo which tend to be replaced by typical migraine after a few years.

Just as with migraine itself, vestibular migraine is diagnosed on the basis of the patient's history. For the diagnosis of migraine, operational criteria have been introduced by the ICHD (Table 4.3).

Migraine *with* aura is less common than migraine *without* aura and includes transient neurological symptoms, each lasting from 5 to 60 minutes, such as scintillating scotoma, wandering unilateral paraesthesia or, rarely, unilateral weakness and aphasia. Visual auras are characterised by bright scintillating lights or zigzag lines, often with a scotoma that interferes with reading. Visual auras typically expand over 5–20 minutes and last for less than 60 minutes. They are often, but not always, restricted to one hemifield. These symptoms usually precede the headache.

Table 4.3 International Classification of Headache Disorders (ICHD) criteria for the diagnosis of migraine without aura

A.	At least five attacks fulfilling B–D
B.	Headache attacks lasting 4–72 hours (untreated or unsuccessfully treated)
C.	Headaches having at least two of the following characteristics: – unilateral location – pulsating quality – moderate or severe pain intensity – aggravation by walking stairs or similar routine physical activity
D.	During headache at least one of the following: – nausea and/or vomiting – photophobia and phonophobia
E.	Not better accounted for by another diagnosis

Table 4.4 Diagnostic criteria for vestibular migraine

A.	At least 5 episodes with vestibular symptoms of moderate or severe intensity, lasting 5 min to 72 hours
B.	Current or previous history of migraine with or without aura according to the International Classification of Headache Disorders (ICHD)
C.	One or more migraine features with at least 50% of the vestibular episodes: – headache with at least two of the following characteristics: one-sided location, pulsating quality, moderate or severe pain intensity, aggravation by routine physical activity – photophobia and phonophobia – visual aura
D.	Not better accounted for by another vestibular or ICHD diagnosis

Table 4.5 Diagnostic criteria for probable vestibular migraine

A.	At least 5 episodes with vestibular symptoms of moderate or severe intensity, lasting 5 min to 72 hours
B.	Only one of the criteria B and C for vestibular migraine is fulfilled (migraine history *or* migraine features during the episode)
C.	Not better accounted for by another vestibular or ICHD diagnosis

Diagnostic criteria for vestibular migraine were included in the International Classification of Headache Disorders (ICHD-III, 2013) in an appendix for new syndromes (Table 4.4).

A separate diagnostic category of *probable* vestibular migraine can be useful for patients who do not entirely fulfil the above criteria but are still considererd to have vestibular migraine as the most likely diagnosis (Table 4.5). Some of them may have headaches that do not correspond fully to the ICHD criteria for migraine or have no headaches at all, while others may have no migraine symptoms during their vertiginous episodes.

Vestibular migraine is quite variable in its clinical presentation. It may manifest itself with spontaneous spinning vertigo, positional vertigo, visually induced or head motion-induced vertigo. These different presentations may occur in isolation, simultaneously or sequentially. Long-lasting attacks over hours or even days may present initially with spinning vertigo that is aggravated by positional change and head movement, turning into pure positional vertigo, head motion-induced dizziness or unsteadiness of decreasing severity later on. Visually induced dizziness is typically triggered by movement of the visual environment (e.g. cinema, traffic, crowds) or by looking at complex visual patterns (e.g. when walking along supermarket aisles or ironing a striped shirt). As with any other vestibular disorder, nausea and imbalance are common accompaniments during the acute phase. The concurrence of migraine symptoms may not be volunteered by the patient and has to be specifically enquired about. Sometimes, prospective recording of symptoms and precipitants (including menstrual cycle) in a dizziness diary can be helpful to direct the patient's attention to specific symptoms and to retrieve the relevant information. Phonophobia is defined as bilateral sound-induced discomfort and must be differentiated from recruitment, which is typically unilateral and persistent. Recruitment leads to an enhanced perception and often distortion of loud sounds in an ear with decreased hearing, e.g. in the late stage of Ménière's disease.

Duration of attacks ranges from a few minutes to several days. Some patients need several weeks to recover fully from an attack. Only 20–30% of patients have attacks lasting between five minutes and one hour as would be expected from a typical migraine aura, while 50–70% have vertigo for hours and days. Some patients experience a series of brief vertiginous spells over a period of several hours on a background of mild to moderate dizziness. This pattern resembles migraines with a mild to moderate baseline headache punctuated by brief attacks of severe stabbing headache.

The temporal association of vertigo and headache varies within and between individuals. Only a minority have migraine headaches as a regular accompaniment to their vertigo, while others have attenuated headaches as compared with their usual ones or have attacks with or without headaches. Some have never experienced the two symptoms together. The symptomatology of migraine may change in individual patients in the course of years. Thus, vestibular migraine may appear long after migraine headaches have ceased. This is why it is critical to enquire about a previous history of headaches and about migraine symptoms other than headache that may accompany the vertigo.

Cochlear symptoms such as hearing loss, tinnitus or aural fullness have been reported in as many as 10–40% of patients with vestibular migraine. Between 10 and 20% develop mild to moderate bilateral downsloping hearing loss, which progresses slowly over the years. About 5% of migraine patients with vestibulo-cochlear symptoms can be diagnosed with Ménière's disease which, according to the above criteria, prohibits a diagnosis of vestibular migraine. However, most patients with vestibular migraine and cochlear symptoms do not meet the criteria for Ménière's disease, since their hearing loss is mild and non-progressive.

About half of the patients with vestibular migraine have comorbid anxiety and depression, which may cause permanent dizziness in between attacks. This so-called persistent perceptual dizziness (see page 135) needs to be recognised and explained to the patient to pave the way for specific treatment.

Clinical examination is usually normal between attacks. Neuro-ophthalmological evaluation may reveal mild central deficits, such as persistent positional nystagmus and saccadic pursuit, particularly in patients with a long history of vestibular migraine. Interictal head-shaking nystagmus occurs in less than 50% of patients. Video-oculographic recordings during the acute attack have shown various types and combinations of spontaneous and persistent positional nystagmus. Most common is a central type of spontaneous nystagmus such as downbeat, upbeat or torsional nystagmus. In addition, or as a solitary finding, patients may have central positional nystagmus which can be suspected when the provoking position and the nystagmus plane do not suggest excitation of a single peripheral semicircular canal (see 'Central positional nystagmus', page 125). A minority of patients have spontaneous horizontal–torsional nystagmus and contralateral hypofunction of the vestibulo-ocular reflex (VOR) consistent with peripheral vestibular loss on that side.

Pathophysiology

The pathophysiology of vestibular migraine is unknown. Short-lasting vertigo, fulfilling the criteria of a migraine aura, has been hypothetically linked to transient hypo-perfusion of the labyrinth. However, aura-related vasoconstriction is usually not severe enough to produce ischaemic symptoms but is rather regarded as a secondary phenomenon.

Trea

Ther:
Many
and r
pharr
such
biofe
30 m
T
far, s
orien
symp
is wo
drug
suppr
side-e
prelir
migra
both
anti-i
M
pharr
Treat
accou
como
reduc
and h
be an
the o!
A
of syr
titrati
each (
tolera
three
of its
when
only i
to 50
up tc
vestib
A
can b
heada
taper(
patiei

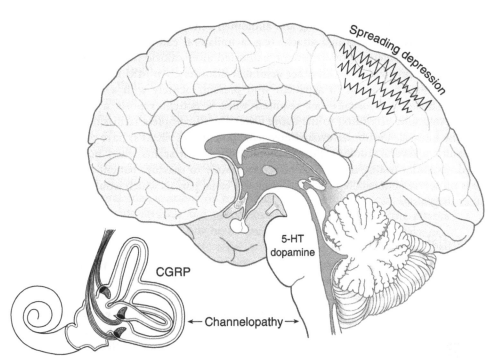

Figure 4.1 Hypothetical mechanisms of vestibular migraine including spreading depression reaching vestibular cortical areas, release of dopamine (or other neurotransmitters) in the vestibular nuclei, release of the neuropeptide CGRP in the vestibular end organs or brainstem, and dysfunctional ion channels affecting labyrinthine, brainstem or cerebellar function.

A spreading wave of depression, which is likely to cause cortical aura symptoms, may produce vertigo when vestibular cortex areas are affected, although the complex nystagmus patterns observed during acute vestibular migraine would not be consistent with a purely cortical mechanism. Another explanation refers to the neurotransmitters released during migraine attacks and which are known to modulate vestibular function; they include noradrenaline, 5-hydroxytryptamine, dopamine and the neuropeptide CGRP. The different sites of action of these transmitters and their varying contributions to individual attacks may explain the clinical variability of vestibular migraine. Another hypothesis relates vestibular migraine to genetic defects of ion channels which have been identified as the cause of several paroxysmal disorders, including periodic paralysis, episodic ataxia and familial hemiplegic migraine. Interestingly, both episodic ataxia and familial hemiplegic migraine often involve migraine headaches and paroxysmal vertigo. Thus, one may speculate that in vestibular migraine a defective ion channel with predominant expression in the brain and inner ear may lead to local ion imbalances, causing transient dysfunction of the labyrinthine sensory organs and central vestibular structures (Figure 4.1). Finally, the proximity and the reciprocal connections between the trigeminal and vestibular nuclei have led to the hypothesis that trigeminal activation during migraine attacks may spread to the vestibular system.

Investigations

Neither migraine nor vestibular migraine can be diagnosed or confirmed by biochemical, neurophysiological or imaging findings. Therefore, the role of such investigations is limited.

Table 4.6 Pharmacological treatment of vestibular migraine

Drug and dose	Common side-effects	Contraindications/precautions
Acute attacks		
Dimenhydrinate 50–100 mg PO or 150 mg supp or IV every 8–12 h	Sedation, dry mouth	Glaucoma, asthma, urinary retention
Diazepam 2–10 mg PO, supp or IV every 6 h	Sedation, lethargy	COPD, respiratory failure, addiction
Sumatriptan 50–100 mg PO, 10–20 mg IN 25 mg supp, 6 mg SC	Chest pain, throat tightness, palpitations, paraesthesia	Coronary artery disease, hypotension, use of ergotamine
Zolmitriptan 2.5–5 mg PO, 5 mg IN	Same as above	Same as above
Rizatriptan 10 mg PO	Same as above	Same as above
Prophylaxis		
Propranolol 40–240 mg/d PO	Bradycardia, bronchospasm, heart block, hypotension, depression, fatigue, cold extremities	COPD, bradycardia, heart block, diabetes, peripheral arterial disease
Metoprolol 100–200 mg/d PO	Same as above	Same as above
Valproic acid 500–2000 mg/d PO	Nausea, weight gain, tremor	Liver disease
Amitriptyline 25–200 mg/d PO	Sedation, hypotension, confusion, dry mouth, rarely cardiac arrhythmia	Arrhythmia, glaucoma, urinary retention, mania
Pizotifen 1.5 mg/d PO	Sedation, dry mouth, weight gain	Glaucoma, urinary retention, obesity
Flunarizine 5–10 mg/d PO	Sedation, weight gain, exacerbation of depression, parkinsonian symptoms	History of depression
Topiramate 50–200 mg/d PO	Delirium, psychosis, weight loss, paraesthesia	Psychiatric disorder

Routes of administration: PO = oral, IV = intravenous, supp = suppository, SC = subcutaneous, IN = intranasal. COPD = chronic obstructive pulmonary disease.

Benign recurrent vertigo

The term *benign recurrent vertigo* has been used to imply a causal relationship with migraine. Some authors have used it to include all varieties of vestibular migraine, while others (including ourselves) restrict it to patients with recurrent vertigo of unknown origin. Indeed, there are patients with isolated recurrent vertigo without any personal history of migraine, migrainous symptoms during the attack or typical triggers, who would not even meet the criteria for probable vestibular migraine. As such attacks can still be caused by a migraine mechanism (just as isolated migraine auras may occur in patients who have never had a typical migraine headache), a trial with prophylactic migraine medication can be justified (Table 4.6), after exclusion of other causes of recurrent vertigo (see Table 4.1, page 70).

Ménière's disease

Table 4.7 Ménière's disease: key features

History	Attacks of spinning vertigo lasting 20 minutes to several hours with unilateral tinnitus, hearing loss and aural fullness Fluctuating hearing loss with recovery in the early stages and progression later on
Clinical findings	Initially normal between attacks; later low-frequency hearing loss on the affected side progressing to a flat pattern
Pathophysiology	Increased pressure within the endolymphatic space (hydrops) leading to mechanical and chemical irritation of the labyrinthine sensory organs
Investigations	Repeated audiometry to document fluctuating low-tone hearing loss in the early stages and then progressive hearing loss Caloric testing may show unilateral canal paresis
Treatment	Vestibular suppressants for acute attacks; evidence for prophylaxis with betahistine, low-salt diet ± diuretics or steroids is weak; intratympanic gentamicin for refractory patients with frequent and severe attacks.

Ménière's disease is characterised by recurrent vertigo with cochlear symptoms. The associated pathology is endolymphatic hydrops, which designates the expansion of the endolymphatic space within the labyrinth. Endolymphatic hydrops can be idiopathic or secondary to inner-ear trauma, infection and metabolic disturbance. Only the (more common) idiopathic variant is called Ménière's disease while identical symptoms from a recognised cause are called Ménière's syndrome.

Ménière's disease is rare but overdiagnosed in our experience. Reported prevalence ranges from 20 to 200 per 100,000 compared to about 1,000 per 100,000 for vestibular migraine. Men and women are affected almost equally. Age at the time of diagnosis is typically between 30 and 60 years. Onset after 70 or before 20 years of age is rare. Familial occurrence has been noted in about 10% of patients.

Clinical features

The hallmarks of Ménière's disease are attacks of vertigo, hearing loss, tinnitus and aural fullness. Often an attack starts with cochlear symptoms, i.e. a roaring or rushing tinnitus, a sensation of aural fullness and hearing loss. Seconds or minutes later vertigo sets in, peaking rapidly in intensity and then declining over the course of 20 minutes to several hours. Common associated features include nausea, vomiting, sweating and imbalance, while diarrhoea occurs in severe attacks only. Often, patients are forced to lie motionless until the spell subsides, as any head movement makes it worse. Afterwards, they may feel unsteady for a day or two. Attacks often start with an excitatory spontaneous nystagmus beating to the involved ear for several minutes, followed by an inhibitory nystagmus beating to the healthy side for several hours. Subsequently, another nystagmus reversal may occur, so-called *recovery nystagmus*.

In the early stages of the disorder vestibular or cochlear symptoms may occur in isolation. After two or three years, however, the complete set of symptoms is usually established. Patients with a long-standing history of recurrent isolated vertigo and no auditory symptoms are therefore unlikely to have Ménière's disease. Some patients may not notice hearing loss during the attack because all attention is focused on the agonising experience of vertigo. In this situation, prospective monitoring of symptoms in a dizziness diary may reveal the full clinical picture. Sometimes, hearing loss occurs without a clear relation to the vertigo attacks. About 50% of the patients experience migraine symptoms, such as headache, phono- and photophobia, during attacks.

Attack frequency varies from several times a week to less than once in a year with unpredictable changes in the course of the disease. Initially, the hearing loss and tinnitus recede fully after an attack. At this stage, audiometric documentation of a fluctuating sensorineural hearing loss, especially in the low-frequency range, may provide essential diagnostic information. Later, a progressive deterioration of hearing is superimposed on the fluctuations and the whole frequency spectrum becomes involved. Similarly, the tinnitus becomes permanent but its intensity may still fluctuate. The end stage (burnt-out phase) of Ménière's disease is reached after about 5–15 years with cessation of episodic vertigo, but there is constant mild disequilibrium, severe permanent hearing loss (but no complete deafness) and unremitting tinnitus on the affected side. Ménière's disease becomes bilateral in about 50% of patients. Involvement of the opposite ear may start during the acute phase of the first year or many years later.

Sudden falls without associated vertigo or loss of consciousness, which have been called *otolithic catastrophes* by Tumarkin, may complicate Ménière's disease at all stages of the disorder. During these episodes patients feel pushed to the ground by some violent external force. Usually, they can get back to their feet immediately afterwards and resume their activities, but some suffer severe injuries including fractures. The presumed mechanism for these attacks is an unstable otolith function leading to unilateral breakdown of vestibulospinal muscle tone. Benign paroxysmal positional vertigo is another complication of Ménière's disease and has been reported in up to 40% of patients.

Delayed endolymphatic hydrops, a variant of Ménière's syndrome, may develop in patients who have had a deaf ear of any cause for many years or even several decades. Interestingly, Ménière symptoms in these patients can affect either the ipsilateral or the contralateral ear suggesting an immunological mechanism of the disorder. With ipsilateral involvement the cochlear symptoms of Ménière's syndrome may be masked by the pre-existing hearing loss. However, aural pressure may point to a hydropic mechanism.

Pathophysiology

Endolymphatic hydrops is an almost universal finding in postmortem studies of patients with Ménière's disease. The cause of this distension of the endolymphatic space is as obscure as the mechanism by which it causes paroxysmal and progressive dysfunction of the inner-ear sensory organs. Hydrops may result from either increased production or decreased resorption of the endolymph. The endolymphatic duct and sac, an appendix of

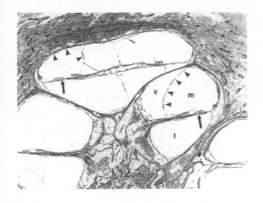

Figure 4.2 Endolymphatic hydrops of the inner ear. Distension of the endolymphatic space (arrowheads) in the cochlea leading to displacement of the organ of Corti (arrows). m = scala media (endolymphatic space), v = scala vestibuli, t = scala tympani. (From: Baloh, Halmagyi, copyright 1996 Oxford University Press Inc., used by permission.)

the endolymphatic space, are known to participate in the resorption of the endolymph. Thus, one speculative mechanism for the development of hydrops implicates obstruction within the endolymphatic duct or sac. This concept is supported by experimental findings in guinea pigs which develop hydrops after ligature of the endolymphatic duct although the same procedure does not lead to endolymphatic hydrops in monkeys. More recent findings indicate that homeostasis of the endolymphatic fluid volume and composition is largely regulated by active ion transport, which raises the possibility that the underlying problem is an ion-channel disorder.

Several hypotheses have been proposed to explain the recurrent and permanent symptoms of Ménière's disease. The traditional view is that rupture of the membranes separating the endolymph from the surrounding perilymph leads to transient hair-cell dysfunction caused by potassium intoxication, because the endolymph is rich in potassium whereas the perilymph is not. Rapid healing of the rupture would then restore the usual ion concentrations. Alternative explanations include mechanical interference of the hydrops with the inner-ear sensory epithelia which is readily visible on pathological specimens (Figure 4.2), pressure-induced compromise of the hair cells' blood supply, and paroxysmal dysfunction of ion channels in labyrinthine hair cells.

Investigations

Ménière's disease is diagnosed by taking a meticulous history, eliciting the typical combination of vestibular and cochlear symptoms and their characteristic temporal profile. Audiometry is useful to document the low-frequency sensorineural hearing loss and fluctuations which are typical for the early stages. Electro-cochleography, which is available in specialised audiology departments, can be useful for patients with an equivocal history and shows a characteristic pattern in the presence of hydrops (elevated ratio of summating potential and nerve action potential). However, the sensitivity of electrocochleography is clearly less than optimal so that some patients with Ménière's disease will be missed. Brainstem auditory-evoked responses (BAER) are usually normal. Electro- or video-oculography may show spontaneous horizontal nystagmus beating either to the involved or to the healthy side, reflecting either an irritative or defective phase of the involved labyrinth. Unilateral hypofunction to caloric irrigation or video head-impulse testing (vHIT) occurs in about half of the patients on the clinically involved side and 20% on the opposite side. Total unilateral loss of function occurs in about 10%.

These findings are non-specific and can occur with most vestibular disorders. Fluctuations of caloric responses with repeated testing is a more specific finding observed in 40% of patients. Cervical vestibular-evoked myogenic potentials (cVEMPs) can be normal, enlarged, decreased or absent in an ear with Ménière's disease; in other words, one would rather not do them. MRI is not strictly necessary for diagnosis. However, as patients will normally have unilateral audio-vestibular abnormalities MRI is advisable for ruling out a structural cerebello-pontine angle lesion. Patients with the clinical features of bilateral Ménière's syndrome should be screened for syphilis (FTA-ABS) and autoimmune inner-ear disease (see page 89).

Differential diagnosis

Symptomatic forms of endolymphatic hydrops producing the typical symptoms of Ménière's disease have been reported after head trauma, with viral, bacterial and syphilitic labyrinthitis and with otosclerosis. The wider differential diagnosis of episodic vertigo with cochlear symptoms unrelated to hydrops includes vertebrobasilar TIA (see page 84), vestibular migraine (page 71), perilymph fistula (page 88), syphilis of the inner ear (page 89), autoimmune inner-ear disease (page 89), vestibular paroxysmia (page 89), acoustic neuroma (page 90) and otosclerosis (page 91). Distinction from Ménière's disease is usually possible on the basis of clinical presentation (Table 4.8).

Table 4.8 Differential diagnosis of Ménière's disease: disorders which may present with vertigo and cochlear symptoms

Diagnosis	Distinctive features
Vertebrobasilar transient ischaemic attacks	Attacks lasting minutes; elderly patients; vascular risk factors; few attacks over weeks or months (rarely years)
Perilymph fistula	Onset often after trauma, strain, barotrauma, cholesteatoma, symptom provocation by pressure changes or loud sounds
Syphilis of the inner ear	Early bilateral involvement; signs of congenital or late acquired syphilis, particularly interstitial keratitis; positive FTA-ABS test
Autoimmune inner-ear disease	Rapid progression and early bilateral involvement; other features of autoimmune disease; autoantibodies may be positive
Vestibular paroxysmia	Brief attacks (seconds), many times per day; mild hearing loss, if any
Acoustic neuroma	Progressive rather than fluctuating hearing loss and tinnitus; usually mild vertigo in < 50% of patients; BAER and MRI abnormal
Otosclerosis	Onset mostly before age of 30 years, auditory symptoms predominate, conductive ± sensorineural hearing loss, usually bilateral
Herpes zoster oticus	Monophasic disorder with unilateral facial palsy, vesicular rash in the auditory canal, ear pain and often unilateral vestibular and hearing loss

BAER = brainstem auditory-evoked response
MRI = magnetic resonance imaging

Treatment

No treatment has been found to halt the progressive destruction of the inner ear in Ménière's disease. However, symptomatic relief can be achieved with oral and transtympanic medication, counselling and (rarely) surgical intervention. First, the nature of the disorder should be openly explained to the patient, forming the basis of a trusting relationship. Unnecessary fears may be relieved when the potential for long asymptomatic intervals and the eventually self-limiting course of the disease are mentioned. Some patients fear that they may go completely deaf, which is wrong for two reasons: the contralateral ear is spared in half of the patients, and residual hearing on the affected side can be useful when combined with a hearing aid. Vestibular rehabilitation is useful both for persistent imbalance, loss of confidence and secondary anxiety observed in many patients (see page 169).

Acute attacks can be alleviated with vestibular suppressants, although nausea or vomiting can interfere with oral administration. Thus, rectal dimenhydrinate (e.g. 150 mg), buccal prochloperazine (3 or 6mg, placed high under the upper lip) and mouth-dissolving lorazepam (1–2 mg) are useful. For further details see Chapter 8. Patients should carry medication with them for attacks away from home. A sick bag and a mobile phone are also helpful in this situation.

Numerous treatments have been advocated for prophylaxis but well-conducted randomised studies are largely lacking. There is no evidence that betahistine (8–16 mg three times a day), favoured in many countries, may reduce attack frequency and severity. It has been advocated that higher doses up to 48 mg three times a day may be more effective, but evidence is missing. Some neuro-otologists start with a low-salt diet, either alone or in combination with a diuretic such as bendrofluazide 2.5 to 5 mg in the morning. The underlying assumption is that this may decrease inner-ear fluid volume. An effective low-salt diet requires a major adaptation in lifestyle with elimination of most processed foods such as salted snacks, canned food, cheese and even ordinary bread, which many patients find unacceptable. Compliance can be supported by repeated dietary counselling and measurement of urine salt excretion which should be below 50 mmol/d but, again, the scientific evidence supporting this approach is meagre. If applied, both betahistine and low-salt/diuretics should be tried for at least two months, with monitoring of symptoms in a diary before their efficacy is assessed. Patients should know that prophylactic treatment will neither prevent nor delay the progression of hearing loss.

When attacks occur at high frequency and intensity for several months, invasive procedures have to be considered. The most effective option is intratympanic instillation of gentamicin, an ototoxic aminoglycoside, or steroids such as methylprednisolone into the middle ear, which can be done during routine outpatient visits in ENT departments. Gentamicin reaches the labyrinth mostly through the round window membrane and exerts its effect primarily on vestibular hair cells, thus allowing preservation of hearing in most patients. Symptoms from the resulting subacute unilateral vestibular loss can be alleviated by vestibular rehabilitation exercises, which can start even before the first treatment session. Gentamicin is also effective to prevent Tumarkin otolithic crises. Intratympanic steroids are a good, non-ablative alternative, with mounting evidence for their efficacy. Endolymphatic sac surgery for Ménière's disease is regarded with scepticism after a controlled trial failed to show any superiority over a sham operation. Labyrinthectomies and vestibular nerve sections are nowadays restricted to the rare patients with severe attacks who do not respond to intratympanic gentamicin or steroid injections.

Vertigo due to vertebrobasilar transient ischaemic attack (TIA)

Table 4.9 Vertiginous transient ischaemic attack: key features

History	Spontaneous attacks of vertigo with abrupt onset lasting minutes, often with other posterior circulation symptoms, e.g. facial numbness, diplopia Affects older adults with vascular risk factors
Clinical findings	Examination may reveal signs of atherosclerosis and of previous cerebral or inner-ear ischaemia, e.g. a carotid bruit, hemiparesis or hearing loss
Pathophysiology	Transient hypoperfusion of the labyrinth, of the vestibular nuclei or cerebellum
Investigations	Audiometry and calorics to search for labyrinthine damage; vascular studies: neck vessel ultrasound, MR-angiography; cerebral angiography in selected patients only
Treatment	Control of risk factors; antiplatelet drugs; rarely stenting of large vessel stenosis

Clinical features

Vertebrobasilar TIA is an infrequent cause of recurrent vertigo. The typical patient with vertigo caused by vertebrobasilar TIA is above 60 years of age and has vascular risk factors such as smoking, hypertension, diabetes or hyperlipidaemia. Heart disease associated with cardiac embolism is an uncommon risk factor since repeated embolisation to the labyrinth or vestibular nuclei is quite unlikely.

Attacks may present with isolated vertigo, but more commonly include associated symptoms from the posterior circulation territory (Table 4.10). Even patients with isolated vertigo tend to have other paroxysmal symptoms from the vertebrobasilar territory on other occasions. Therefore, when a patient presents with recurrent isolated vertigo over an extended period (more than six months), the diagnosis of vertebrobasilar TIA is unconvincing. Vertigo caused by vertebrobasilar TIA occurs spontaneously and starts abruptly. The duration of TIAs has been arbitrarily limited to 24 hours, but the majority last minutes or one to two hours. Attacks lasting more than a few hours usually lead to cerebral infarction visible on MRI which has made the 24-hour limit for TIAs doubtful. Ischaemic vertigo is only rarely provoked by turning or extending the neck. Most neck-movement-related vertigo is in fact *head*-movement-related, reflecting vestibular disease such as benign positional vertigo or poorly compensated unilateral vestibular loss. (For details of cervical and head-extension vertigo, see Chapter 5, page 128.)

Clinical examination may reveal signs of vascular disease such as decreased pulses or bruits over large arteries. Previously unrecognised infarctions may be disclosed by neurological signs such as mental slowing, asymmetric reflexes, Babinski's sign, visual field defects, oculomotor abnormalities or unilateral hearing loss. Vertebrobasilar TIAs may concur with other vascular syndromes causing vertigo or imbalance, such as previous brainstem strokes or cerebral small-vessel disease (see page 152).

Pathophysiology

The posterior circulation supplies both central and peripheral parts of the vestibular system. The posterior inferior cerebellar artery (PICA) originates from the vertebral arteries and irrigates the caudal cerebellum and the lateral medulla, including the caudal portion of the

Table 4.10 Associated symptoms in 42 patients with vertigo due to vertebrobasilar disease

Symptom	Patients
Visual (diplopia, field defects)	29
Drop attacks	14
Unsteadiness, incoordination	9
Extremity weakness	9
Confusion	7
Headache	6
Hearing loss	6
Loss of consciousness	4
Extremity numbness	4
Dysarthria	4
Tinnitus	4
Perioral numbness	2

Source: Grad, Baloh. 1989.

vestibular nuclei. The anterior inferior cerebellar artery (AICA) branches from the basilar artery to supply the mid-portion of the cerebellum and the lateral pons with the rostral portion of the vestibular nuclei, the vestibular nerve and the labyrinth. Therefore, vertigo caused by vertebrobasilar ischaemia may originate either from the labyrinth or from the brainstem. Arguments favouring the labyrinth as the usual source of ischaemic vertigo include the small calibre of the labyrinthine arteries and the common association of vascular vertigo with unilateral canal paresis and a cochlear type of hearing loss.

Transient ischaemia of vestibular structures may result from various mechanisms, e.g. small-vessel occlusion, arterio-arterial emboli, large-vessel stenosis with or without super-imposed thrombosis and arterial dissection. In contrast, cardiac emboli usually affect various territories and are rather unlikely in patients with recurrent vertigo. Spondylotic compression of the vertebral artery leading to vertebrobasilar hypoperfusion on extreme head rotations, so-called rotational vertebral artery occlusion syndrome, has been documented angiographically but is probably very rare.

Investigations

Audiometry and vestibular testing are useful to document permanent damage to the labyrinth or to central pathways. Doppler ultrasound studies can identify narrowing or occlusion of large extra- and intracranial vessels, whereas MRI or CT angiography can also visualise medium-sized vessels. Digital subtraction angiography should be considered when arterial dissection is suspected, which is not sufficiently visualised on MR or CT angiography. Transoesophageal echocardiography may help in selected patients to identify cardiac thrombi or plaques and thrombi in the aortic arch, a frequent source of emboli to the posterior circulation.

Differential diagnosis

When an elderly patient with vascular risk factors presents with unprovoked attacks of vertigo lasting minutes and associated transient symptoms from the posterior circulation (see Table 4.10), the diagnosis is straightforward. The only alternative diagnosis would be migraine with brainstem aura, which likewise involves vertebrobasilar symptoms, but which rarely starts late in life. Therefore, one should enquire about a history of migraine and migrainous symptoms accompanying the vertigo. When vertigo concurs with auditory but no other symptoms various labyrinthine disorders have to be considered (see Tables 4.1 and 4.8). Isolated and unprovoked recurrent vertigo for more than six months is hardly compatible with an underlying vascular disorder and is most commonly related to migraine (see page 71).

Treatment

Both doctor and patient have to take responsibility for correction of vascular risk factors. The risk for cerebral infarction after TIA is 10–15% within 90 days. The risk goes up to 22% for TIA patients who have vertebrobasilar stenosis of more than 50% documented by angiography. Antiplatelet drugs such as aspirin or clopidogrel reduce the relative risk for subsequent cerebral infarction by 18%. Oral anticoagulation is not superior to aspirin in patients with TIAs caused by intracranial stenosis. Statins are effective for lowering the associated risk for myocardial infarction, but have only minimal potential in the secondary prevention of strokes. Angioplasty is increasingly employed to treat vertebral and basilar stenosis. However, the rate of early strokes (within 30 days) seems to be elevated in comparison to medically managed patients. Controlled trials of sufficient size are still lacking to assess the long-term risks and benefits of this procedure.

Vestibular paroxysmia: vascular compression of the eighth nerve?

Some patients with recurrent vertigo and/or oscillopsia have very brief attacks lasting just a few seconds or a minute, often recurring many times per day. Unfortunately, clinical evaluation during an attack is rarely possible and patients are normal during the interval. Neurosurgeons have introduced the concept of *neurovascular compression of the eighth nerve,* an analogy to well-defined cranial nerve syndromes such as trigeminal neuralgia and hemifacial spasm, and have reported good response to surgical decompression of the nerve. They coined the term 'disabling positional vertigo', under the impression that many of these patients had a strong positional component to the vertigo. However, case series on the syndrome have been criticised for their lack of reliable diagnostic criteria and the insufficient exclusion of other disorders causing vertigo, including benign paroxysmal positional vertigo. Sensitivity to positional change is a controversial aspect because it has not been well documented with nystagmus recordings. In addition, positional precipitation of attacks is not a usual feature of other neurovascular compression syndromes such as trigeminal neuralgia and hemifacial spasm. Furthermore, MRI and postmortem studies have shown that asymptomatic contacts between vessels and the eighth nerve can be found in more than 20% of healthy individuals. Therefore, even the radiological finding of a neurovascular contact does not confirm the diagnosis. Several

Table 4.11 Proposed diagnostic criteria for vestibular paroxysmia: neurovascular compression of the eighth nerve. A diagnosis of definite vestibular paroxysmia requires four core criteria or three core criteria and an additional criterion.

Core criteria:

Short attacks of vertigo lasting for seconds to a few minutes

Imbalance during attacks

Attacks occur at rest or are provoked by hyperventilation or particular head positions

No central ocular motor disorder

Response to carbamazepine

Additional criteria:

Hearing loss or tinnitus, permanently or during the attack

Auditory or vestibular deficits measurable by neurophysiological methods

Source: Hüfner, Barresi, Glaser et al. 2008.

case reports have demonstrated that paroxysmal nystagmus may be caused also by intra-axial brainstem lesions.

On the other hand, the concept of symptomatic vascular compression of the eighth nerve is supported by the concurrence of paroxysmal vestibulo-cochlear symptoms in patients with established neurovascular compression syndromes such as hemifacial spasm. A neurovascular compression of the neighbouring seventh and eighth cranial nerves has been found intra-operatively in several of these patients. Brandt and Dieterich termed the condition *vestibular paroxysmia* and reported a series of patients with short attacks of vertigo, often precipitated by head movements. Usually, patients responded to treatment with carbamazepine. In a follow-up study most patients reported both spontaneous and provoked attacks, e.g. by turning the head. Hyperventilation-induced nystagmus was observed in 70% of the patients while 60% had unilateral caloric weakness. Neurovascular contacts of the eighth cranial nerve were identified in all but one patient on MRI using so-called CISS sequences (Table 4.11). However, before ordering an MRI, one should remember that neurovascular contacts are found in 20–30% of asymptomatic individuals.

The differential diagnosis of brief attacks of vertigo includes benign paroxysmal positional vertigo (see page 109), vestibular migraine (page 71), benign paroxysmal vertigo of childhood, a childhood variant of vestibular migraine (page 72), episodic ataxia type 2 (page 92) and paroxysmal attacks in multiple sclerosis and other brainstem disorders. Short attacks provoked by changes of middle-ear pressure or loud sounds point to a perilymph fistula or superior canal dehiscence (see page 89), while brief spells elicited by head movement may indicate poorly compensated unilateral vestibular loss (see page 91). In Ménière's disease, very brief attacks may appear in addition to the longer attacks lasting 20 minutes to several hours that are required to make the diagnosis.

For practical purposes, one should try carbamazepine in patients who present with brief attacks of vertigo several times per day after these differential diagnoses have been considered and no cause has been found. In case of failure this may be followed by a migraine prophylactic agent. Surgical decompression may be rarely justified in severely affected patients who are resistant to drug treatment, when MRI visualises a vessel displacing the nerve.

Perilymph fistula

Perilymph fistulas result from a defect in the bony capsule of the labyrinth or in the round or oval windows. Fistulas may be congenital or can be caused by trauma, heavy straining, surgery or diseases eroding the bony labyrinth (Table 4.12). Identification of the event producing the fistula is usually evident from the history. So-called *spontaneous fistulas* are a controversial issue, supposedly originating from straining or minor trauma on the background of a pre-existing subclinical abnormality such as local thinning of the labyrinthine capsule (e.g. superior canal dehiscence syndrome, see below).

Perilymph fistulas related to trauma or straining often start with an audible pop in the affected ear followed by vertigo and hearing loss of any degree. Tinnitus and aural fullness may also occur. Most patients have both auditory and vestibular symptoms but a monosymptomatic course is also possible. Vertigo may be episodic with attacks lasting seconds to days, or chronic with superimposed fluctuations. Once established, a fistula may be sensitive to pressure changes induced by coughing, sneezing or poking the finger into the ear. Some patients experience exacerbations with positional change. The Tullio phenomenon designates provocation of vertigo, oscillopsia and nystagmus by loud sounds and can be related to a fistula due to bony dehiscence of the superior canal. Fistula symptoms may mimic Ménière's disease, but onset immediately after straining, barotrauma or head trauma favours a diagnosis of perilymph fistula.

Clinical examination may reveal decreased hearing, spontaneous nystagmus and unilateral vestibular hypofunction which can be further investigated by audiometry and ENG. The hearing loss is either conductive or sensorineural. Inspection of the ear is mandatory to detect cholesteatoma or other local pathology. A positive fistula test designates the provocation of nystagmus with pressure changes, applied with a finger or a pneumatic otoscope to the ear canal.

To test for a fistula, the patient should also perform a Valsalva manoeuvre (which increases intracranial pressure) while eyes are observed by close inspection, Frenzel's glasses or video-oculography. Syphilis serology is useful in patients with suspected fistula of unknown origin. Thinly sliced CT (0.5 mm to 1 mm) may help to identify bony abnormalities of the labyrinth.. Middle-ear exploration is sometimes performed to identify a leak but often results in equivocal and false-positive findings.

In the patient with an acute fistula, such as after straining, conservative treatment is often advised and includes bed-rest with the head elevated for up to one week, followed by another six weeks during which all straining should be avoided. However, this approach is pragmatic rather than evidence-based. Surgical repair can be attempted in patients refractory to conservative treatment and those with cholesteatoma, acute barotrauma, and penetrating injuries.

Table 4.12 Causes of perilymph fistula

Type	Examples
Congenital	Inner-ear dysplasia, superior canal dehiscence
Trauma	Slap on the ear, explosion, scuba diving, perforating injury to the ear
Straining	Childbirth, weight-lifting, violent sneezing
Surgery	Stapes surgery, other ear surgery
Erosive disease	Cholesteatoma, syphilis, tumour

Rare causes of recurrent vertigo

Superior canal dehiscence

Superior canal dehiscence syndrome has been delineated as a variant of perilymphatic fistula that causes peculiar symptoms and is amenable to treatment. Dehiscence designates not a proper fistula but rather a thinning or discontinuity of the bone that separates the superior canal from the middle cranial fossa. The main symptoms are sound- and pressure-induced vertigo and oscillopsia, while chronic disequilibrium occurs only in a few patients. About 50% of patients have autophony, i.e. they hear their own voice unusually loud, hear their heartbeat, and sometimes even hear their eye movements. Loud sounds applied to the affected ear, a Valsalva manoeuvre against pinched nostrils, or tragus compression evoke a short bout of vertigo. Concomitantly, there is a slow eye movement upward with a torsional component to the contralateral side, which can be best observed under Frenzel's glasses or by video-oculography.

The most important diagnostic procedure is a high-resolution (0.5 mm) temporal bone CT to visualise the bony defect at the apex of the superior canal. Vestibular-evoked myogenic potentials (VEMPs), a test of vestibulo-cervical function available in specialised centres, may be helpful. They can be elicited at a lower threshold than normal in these patients and show enlarged amplitudes, reflecting an increased excitability of the labyrinth due to a third mobile window (in addition to the round and oval windows). The audiogram may show an air–bone gap (due to the fact that patients can hear excessively through the bone). Many patients can avoid activities that provoke symptoms and do not require surgery. However, refractory patients can be treated with surgical resurfacing and plugging of the superior canal.

Autoimmune inner-ear disease

The hallmark of autoimmune inner-ear disease is bilateral, rapidly progressive hearing loss, paired with recurrent vertigo in about 50% of patients. Some patients have isolated vestibular symptoms. Only about 25% have systemic connective tissue disease including lupus erythematosus, Sjögren syndrome, rheumatoid arthritis or vasculitis such as polyarteritis nodosa, Behçet's disease, or Wegener granulomatosis. Cogan's syndrome represents a more localised vasculitis with predominant interstitial keratitis (red eyes) and inner-ear involvement. When no systemic features are present the term *idiopathic bilateral progressive sensorineural hearing loss* is often used. For diagnosis, serial audiograms every few weeks or months are necessary to document the progression of hearing loss. Serological tests for a systemic disorder include antinuclear antibodies (elevated in about 60%) and rheumatoid factor (20%), whereas other markers are rarely helpful. Specific inner-ear antibodies, such as heat-shock protein 70, have been largely abandoned because of insufficient sensitivity and specificity. A response to moderate-dose corticosteroids (e.g. prednisolone 1 mg/kg daily for four weeks followed by tapering) supports the diagnosis of autoimmune inner-ear disease but can be expected in fewer than 50% of patients. Methotrexate and cyclophosphamide have been used as therapeutic alternatives, but a randomised trial with methotrexate failed to show any benefit.

Syphilis of the inner ear

This may occur as a manifestation of early-acquired, late-acquired and late congenital syphilis. In early-acquired syphilis, vestibular symptoms and bilateral hearing loss are caused by meningitis with eighth-nerve involvement. More common is syphilitic osteitis of the temporal bone with associated labyrinthitis and secondary endolymphatic hydrops as a late manifestation of either congenital or acquired syphilis, usually starting between the fourth and sixth decade. Similar to autoimmune inner-ear disease, both late congenital and acquired inner-ear syphilis present with episodic vertigo and fluctuating hearing loss that becomes bilateral within months. The stigmata of congenital syphilis (interstitial keratitis, saddle nose, frontal bossing, Hutchinson's teeth) and signs of tertiary syphilis may provide diagnostic clues. Serological confirmation is based on a positive fluorescent treponema antibody absorption test (FTA-ABS). The CSF is usually normal with syphilitic labyrinthitis, except for patients with concurrent neurosyphilis. Progression to bilateral deafness can often be prevented by combined treatment with penicillin (weekly intramuscular benzathine penicillin, 2.4 million U for three months) and steroids (oral prednisone, 60 mg on alternating days for three to six months, followed by slow tapering).

Schwannoma of the eighth nerve (vestibular/acoustic neuroma)

Vestibular schwannoma rarely causes isolated recurrent vertigo but rather progressive unilateral hearing loss and constant tinnitus. Therefore, schwannoma should be considered primarily when a vertiginous patient has additional hearing loss or tinnitus, particularly when hearing loss is progressive rather than fluctuating (as in Ménière's disease) and when high frequencies are affected most. Vertigo occurs in about 50% of patients with schwannoma of the eighth nerve, often only once in the course of the disease or at long intervals. Its intensity is usually mild to moderate and it is rarely associated with nausea. Duration varies from seconds to hours. The seemingly paradoxical combination of total nerve destruction and only mild vestibular symptoms can be explained by the slow growth of these tumours which allows continuous central compensation of the increasing peripheral deficit. Large tumours usually cause constant disequilibrium due to compression of the caudal cerebellum and dysfunction of the adjacent fifth and seventh cranial nerves. Quite often, nystagmus can be elicited with hyperventilation, beating towards the affected ear when the tumour is small (excitatory nystagmus) and to the opposite side when the tumour is large (lesional nystagmus). BAERs are useful for screening patients with both vertigo and auditory symptoms for vestibular schwannoma. Small tumours ($<$ 2mm) may be missed by BAERs but are often managed with a 'wait and see' strategy anyway. Thus, careful follow-up can be an option when MRI is not readily accessible. MRI typically shows a tumour that stretches from the internal acoustic meatus to the cerebellopontine angle (Figure 4.3). Rarely, other lesions of the cerebello-pontine angle may mimic vestibular schwannoma; examples are a giant aneurysm, meningioma, chordoma, lipoma and epidermoid cyst.

Vestibular epilepsy

Cortical areas that process vestibular information are widely distributed over the hemispheres but the core region of the vestibular cortex is located at the temporoparietal junction and the adjacent posterior insula. Focal epileptic discharges in these areas may provoke rotational vertigo, other illusory motion, gaze deviation, nystagmus and nausea. The typical duration of focal seizures is 30 seconds to 3 minutes. Diagnosis is facilitated when there are other features of simple partial seizures (e.g. a sensory march or an auditory aura) or of complex partial seizures (clouded consciousness, automatisms) resulting from spread of epileptic activity to neighbouring areas, or when secondary generalisation occurs. Electro-encephalography and

A 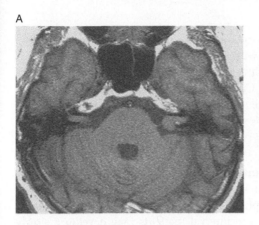 B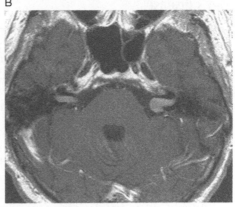

Figure 4.3 **Schwannoma of the eighth nerve** (acoustic neuroma) on the left before (A) and after (B) gadolinium contrast application.

MRI are helpful to document functional and morphological abnormalities in these regions. Treatment includes anticonvulsants that are effective for partial seizures, such as carbamaze-pine, valproate, lamotrigine or levetiracetam. Warning – this is a rare condition. The authors have seen only one convincing case in their combined experience.

Insufficient compensation of unilateral vestibular loss

Most patients with chronic unilateral loss of vestibular function are not vertiginous because, in the process of central compensation, they have learned to control balance and eye movements with only one functioning vestibular organ. Rapid head turns to the affected side, however, may still cause oscillopsia (apparent motion of the environment) and a brief vertiginous sensation. Conversely, when a patient presents with short attacks of vertigo provoked by head movement it is useful to enquire about a previous episode of vestibular neuritis (see page 54) or other preceding inner-ear disease. The second step would be clinical examination of the vestibulo-ocular reflex (head-impulse test, see page 36) and testing for spontaneous or head-shaking nystagmus with Frenzel's glasses, followed by caloric testing. Benign paroxysmal positional vertigo, which may be secondary to vestibular neuritis (see page 59), should be excluded by Hallpike positional testing. Vestibular rehabilitation may help to promote central compensation even at late stages (see page 169).

Otosclerosis

This is a hereditary disorder that leads to bone resorption and new bone formation in the middle and inner ear, starting between the second and fourth decade of life. Otosclerosis is characterised by bilateral, slowly progressive hearing loss of a mixed conductive and sensorineural type. About 20% of patients have vertigo or imbalance due to deformation and destruction of the labyrinthine sensory organs and nerves. A subgroup develops endolymphatic hydrops and has typical Ménière symptoms. The key to diagnosis is the audiogram, which shows a predominantly conductive hearing loss. Hearing can be improved by tympanoplasty while vestibular symptoms may improve with vestibular rehabilitation (see Chapter 8) or treatment of suspected endolymphatic hydrops.

Paget's disease

This is another metabolic disorder of bone resorption with consecutive new bone formation. It usually manifests itself in the sixth decade with a male to female preponderance of 4:1. Paget's disease may affect a single bone or multiple bones, most commonly involving deformation of skull, vertebrae, pelvis, femur and tibia. Conductive and sensorineural hearing loss are common inner-ear symptoms, while progressive unsteadiness and recurrent vertigo are rather rare. Treatment options include bisphosphonates and calcitonin for symptomatic patients.

Episodic ataxia type 2

This is a rare calcium-channel disorder with autosomal dominant inheritance which starts during childhood or adolescence. Attacks of ataxia, often accompanied by vertigo, nausea and headache, are provoked by emotional or physical stress and last in the order of hours. Many patients suffer from migraine also. In the interval, patients may develop a slowly progressive cerebellar syndrome with gaze-evoked or downbeat nystagmus and persistent unsteadiness. Attacks usually respond well to acetazolamide or 4-amino-pyridine. Familial hemiplegic migraine is a closely related inherited disorder which is caused by mutations within the same calcium-channel gene. Attacks are characterised by headache, hemiplegia and often vertigo. Attacks may be prevented by migraine prophylaxis or acetazolamide.

Bilateral vestibulopathy

Idiopathic bilateral vestibulopathy is characterised by constant disequilibrium and oscillopsia during head movements, which develops insidiously over the years (see page 141). However, some patients experience isolated attacks of spinning vertigo lasting seconds or minutes in the early phase of the disease.

What to do if you don't have a clue

Every dizziness specialist sees patients with recurrent vertigo for whom a diagnosis cannot be readily made even after the diagnoses presented above have been considered. The diagnosis may be particularly difficult when there are no precipitants of and accompaniments to the vertigo and when all laboratory investigations are negative. The following considerations and measures can help to handle the situation.

Is it really vertigo?

Many dizzy patients find it difficult to describe their abnormal sensations and jump at any term suggested by their doctor. (Spinning? – Yes, I think so.) Remember that true vertigo usually involves more than just a spinning sensation in the head, but often a spinning of the environment, imbalance, nausea and head motion discomfort. One should be aware, however, that a patient with panic attacks may even report an illusion of the room spinning around, which may be misleading. When the starting point is recurrent dizziness rather than recurrent vertigo another list of differential diagnoses has to be worked up (see Table 4.13, page 93).

Vertigo diary

The diagnosis of vertigo syndromes is mainly based on the recognition of type, combination, precipitation and duration of symptoms. Retrieval of these details from the patient's memory is sometimes not possible since all the patient's attention may have been absorbed by the dreadful experience of vertigo and catastrophic fears. Prospective monitoring of symptoms in a dizziness diary usually helps to ascertain frequency and what really happens during an attack.

Is it vestibular migraine?

The most common diagnosis in patients with isolated recurrent vertigo is vestibular migraine, even in the absence of a migraine history or migrainous symptoms during the attacks. Migraine features may appear later in the course of the disease, thus confirming the diagnosis. Another support (but not proof) for the diagnosis is response to acute or prophylactic antimigraine agents, which can be tried, whenever symptoms are severe enough to warrant pharmacological intervention.

Is it early Ménière's disease?

Ménière's disease sometimes starts with a period of isolated recurrent vertigo which can last up to several years, although isolated fluctuating hearing loss is more common in the early stages. Remember that Ménière attacks last 20 minutes to several hours and that audiometry is useful to detect subclinical hearing loss.

Is it vestibular paroxysmia?

Very short attacks of vertigo lasting seconds may result from vascular compression of the eighth nerve, but the diagnosis is difficult to confirm. In this situation, carbamazepine should be tried as it often relieves this type of vertigo (see page 86).

Should you treat the patient in the absence of a definite diagnosis?

Yes! Provided you have made a serious effort to identify the underlying cause and the patient feels that attacks are frequent and severe enough to warrant treatment, you can try preventive treatment with migraine prophylaxis or carbamazepine. The order will vary with your clinical judgement on the underlying mechanism.

RECURRENT DIZZINESS

Table 4.13 Recurrent dizziness: diagnoses with key features (for recurrent vertigo see page 70)

Disorder	Key features
Orthostatic hypotension (page 94)	Brief episodes of dizziness lasting seconds (to minutes) after standing up; relieved by sitting/lying down; drop of systolic blood pressure of ≥ 20 mmHg after standing up
Cardiac arrhythmia (page 97)	Dizziness lasting seconds; may be accompanied by palpitations; can be caused by bradycardia < 40/min or tachycardia > 170/min
Panic attacks (page 99)	Variable duration from minutes to hours Often provoked by specific situations such as leaving the house, riding on buses or driving, supermarkets, height, crowds, escalators Accompanied by choking, palpitations, tremor, body warmth, anxiety
Drug-induced dizziness (page 102)	Variable clinical presentation according to pharmacological mechanism: sedation, vestibular suppression, ototoxicity, cerebellar toxicity, orthostatic hypotension, hypoglycaemia
Other rare causes (page 106)	Hypertensive crisis, metabolic disorders, height vertigo

Orthostatic hypotension

Table 4.14 Orthostatic hypotension: key features

History	Brief episodes of dizziness lasting seconds (to minutes) after assuming an upright posture; relieved by sitting/lying down; may be followed by syncope Risk factors: old age, dehydration, heat, carbohydrate meals, prolonged bed-rest, various drugs
Clinical findings	Drop of systolic blood pressure of $\geq$ 20 mmHg after standing up, accompanied by dizziness or fainting
Pathophysiology	Often multifactorial: autonomic failure, volume depletion, vasodilatation, associated anaemia Reflex mechanism in neurally mediated syncope
Investigations	Orthostatic blood pressure; heart rate variability; sometimes other autonomic function tests including tilt-table
Treatment	Elimination of offending drugs; increased salt and fluid intake; frequent small meals; head and trunk elevation at night; fludrocortisone, midodrine, erythropoetin
	Patient education (raise slowly); orthostatic training for neurally mediated syncope

Clinical features

Dizziness after standing up due to orthostatic hypotension is probably the most common type of dizziness, with a lifetime prevalence of 13%. It may have severe consequences, causing syncope in 19% and traumatic injury in 5% of affected individuals. Orthostatic hypotension occurs in two different clinical contexts: autonomic failure and neurally mediated syncope. With autonomic failure, orthostatic intolerance is permanent and manifests itself immediately after standing up; whereas with neurally mediated (vasovagal) syncope it is a paroxysmal event, occurring during prolonged upright stance which often requires an additional trigger.

Symptoms are similar in both conditions: warmth, abdominal discomfort, light-headedness, inability to concentrate, blackening or fading out of vision, ringing of the ears or hearing loss and eventually syncope. Pallor and sweating may be associated. The whole sequence can evolve within a few seconds or may take one or two minutes and can be reversed by sitting or lying down. When syncope occurs, the circulatory origin of the preceding dizziness is obvious, but many patients experience only the presyncopal stage of orthostatic hypotension.

Orthostatic intolerance becomes more prevalent with advancing age, affecting between 5 and 30% of older adults. Apart from age-related degeneration of the autonomic system, specific neurological disorders, such as pure autonomic failure, multiple-system atrophy, advanced Parkinson's disease and diabetic neuropathy, compromise autonomic function in older adults. Orthostatic hypotension is aggravated by several factors which may cause orthostatic symptoms even in the absence of autonomic failure, particularly when occurring in combination, such as bed-rest, fever and

Table 4.15 Factors causing or aggravating orthostatic hypotension

Salt/volume depletion

Prolonged bed-rest

Fever

Heat

Hyperventilation

Drugs (diuretics, vasodilators, antihypertensives, dopaminergics, anticholinergics, antidepressants, opiates)

Anaemia

Bilateral carotid stenosis

Table 4.16 Typical triggers for neurally mediated syncope

Prolonged standing

Warm environment

Emotions of fear/helplessness

Sight of blood or injection needle

Venipuncture or any other invasive medical procedure

Sudden pain

Micturition

volume depletion (Table 4.15). In some patients, orthostatic symptoms are most prominent after meals. The neurally mediated variant of orthostatic intolerance affects all age groups and can often be recognised by specific circumstances triggering an acute fall in blood pressure, such as prolonged standing or venipuncture (Table 4.16).

Postural tachycardia syndrome is a variant of orthostatic hypotension with increases of heart rate up to 120–170 beats per minute while standing. Patients complain of orthostatic symptoms such as poor concentration and light-headedness but usually have either normal or only slightly reduced orthostatic blood pressure. Concurrent hyperventilation leading to cerebral vasoconstriction may explain this discrepancy to some extent.

Pathophysiology

Maintenance of cerebral perfusion during upright stance depends critically on peripheral vasoconstriction mediated by sympathetic nerve fibres and on cerebral autoregulation. The efficacy of both of these mechanisms declines with advancing age and may be compromised under specific circumstances even in younger individuals (see Table 4.15). In neurally mediated syncope, the drop in blood pressure usually follows a prolonged period of standing during which blood is pooled in the legs. The ensuing decreased venous return to the heart or specific triggers provoke a reflexive cessation of sympathetic tone with peripheral vasodilatation. This reflex has probably developed during evolution to increase chances for survival after severe blood loss. The sudden drop in blood pressure reduces bleeding while syncope brings the body to a horizontal position, ensuring brain perfusion at low blood pressure levels.

Dizziness due to orthostatic hypotension is usually not related to ischaemia of the labyrinth but rather to widespread cortical hypoperfusion. This results in impaired processing of sensory signals for spatial orientation, diminished attention and cognition and eventually loss of consciousness. Some patients, however, report spinning vertigo prior to fainting, which may result from asymmetric perfusion of the labyrinths.

Investigations

Measurement of orthostatic blood pressure immediately after standing up from supine and then repeatedly for five minutes should be a routine investigation in elderly dizzy patients and in anyone complaining of orthostatic dizziness. A fall of greater than 20 mmHg in systolic blood pressure or greater than 10 mmHg in diastolic blood pressure is regarded as relevant, particularly when accompanied by typical symptoms. Orthostatic hypotension can go unrecognised when measurements are made at times that do not correspond to the patient's usual symptomatic periods, which are often in the morning or after meals.

A *hyper*tensive blood pressure at rest does not argue against a diagnosis of orthostatic *hypo*tension. On the contrary: orthostatic hypotension is most prevalent in elderly patients treated for hypertension. Moreover, patients with autonomic failure often have supine hypertension. Observation of the heart rate during orthostatic testing provides further clues, with a fixed frequency pointing to an underlying disorder of the autonomic nervous system. Extended autonomic testing is only rarely required. In patients with neurocardiogenic syncope, a prolonged orthostatic challenge on a tilt table can prove the propensity to circulatory collapse. When there is a typical history of situation-specific fainting or near fainting, tilt-table testing is not necessary.

Differential diagnosis

Orthostatic dizziness can be readily identified from the patient's history. It should be easily distinguished from positional vertigo which depends on head position with respect to gravity and not on body posture. Thus, positional vertigo may appear after sitting up from lying but not after standing up from sitting with the head kept upright (see Figure 2.1, page 23). Also, positional vertigo is usually present in supine positions whereas orthostatic hypotension is relieved by lying down. Orthostatic symptoms with normal orthostatic blood pressure have been noted with hyperventilation (see page 101) and with the postural tachycardia syndrome (page 95).

Treatment

The first step is reduction or replacement of drugs that interfere with orthostatic tolerance. An equally important measure is increase of salt (extra 3 g to 6 g) and fluid intake (3 to 4 l per day) unless the patient has heart failure. Drinking 500 ml water after awakening raises orthostatic blood pressure by about 30 mmHg! Doctors should invest some time to explain non-pharmacological measures to patients and spouses. Patient education starts with simple advice on how to get up from bed: sit up, wait a minute, stand up and go. Warm environments and straining, which impairs venous return to the heart, should be avoided. Sleeping with the head and trunk elevated by 20° to 30° prevents supine hypertension and nocturnal pressure-natriuresis, thus preserving plasma volume. Regular exercise, such as walking or climbing stairs, has been shown to improve orthostatic tolerance. Dizziness during upright stance can be often prevented by crossing and tensing the legs, which elevated blood pressure by 13% in one study. Waist-high custom-made compression stockings can be very effective, but are often not well tolerated. Hypertensive patients with concurrent orthostatic hypotension should stay upright during the day and take anti-hypertensives only at night. When postprandial hypotension is the predominant problem, frequent small meals of low-carbohydrate content are helpful. Alcohol should be minimised while salt and fluid intake should be increased. Caffeine was ineffective in a controlled trial.

Pharmacological intervention is necessary when behavioural measures fail, even though evidence from controlled trials is weak to date. The alpha-1 adrenergic agonist midodrine (2.5 to 10 mg, two or three times per day, avoid bedtime dose) and fludrocortisone (0.1 mg/d starting dose, followed by weekly increases of 0.1 mg/d up to 0.5 mg/d) are thought to be most effective. Recombinant erythropoietin is useful for patients with autonomic failure and anaemia (4000 U subcutaneously, twice a week for six weeks).

Neurally mediated syncope can often be prevented by reassuring the patient about the benign nature of the disorder and explanation of mechanisms and contributing factors. When possible, the patient should lie down with the legs elevated at the onset of symptoms. Alternatively, physical measures, e.g. by crossing the legs and tensing leg, buttock and abdominal muscles may avert the impending faint. Beta-blockers have been advocated for prevention, but several well-conducted trials have been negative. A cardiac pacemaker is only recommended for patients with frequent asystolic syncope. Orthostatic training, which requires standing with the back against a wall for 30 minutes daily, with feet closed and 15 cm away from the wall were proposed for prevention of neurally mediated syncope. However, results of controlled trials were inconsistent; only motivated patients with a predominantly vasodepressor response on tilt-table testing seem to respond.

Cardiac arrhythmia

Table 4.17 Cardiac arrhythmia: key features

History	Episodes with light-headedness lasting seconds (to minutes), sometimes with palpitations; may evolve to syncope Often history of heart disease
Clinical findings	Either normal in the interval or clinical signs of heart disease
Pathophysiology	Both bradycardia (< 40/min) and tachycardia (> 170/min) may interfere with adequate perfusion of the brain
Investigations	Electrocardiogram; Holter monitoring; rarely invasive electro-physiological testing or implantable loop recorders
Treatment	Correction of metabolic or electrolyte disturbances; antiarrhythmic drugs; cardiac pacemaker; implantable cardioverter defibrillator; radio-frequency ablation

Clinical features

Dizziness related to paroxysmal cardiac arrhythmia is characterised by brief attacks lasting seconds rather than minutes. Prolonged dizziness due to persistent arrhythmia is uncommon. The sensation of dizziness is of a presyncopal type with light-headedness, faintness and associated symptoms such as dimming and blackening out of vision, bilateral tinnitus or hearing loss and eventually syncope. Suggestive features of arrhythmia-related dizziness include palpitations, angina and dyspnoea. Unlike orthostatic hypotension, cardiac arrhythmia may occur with any position of the body. The patient's previous history may reveal an underlying cardiac disorder, a general medical disorder promoting arrhythmia (e.g. thyrotoxicosis, electrolyte imbalance) or arrhythmogenic drugs (e.g. tricyclics, antiarrhythmics). Clinical examination focuses on pulse rate and rhythm, central–peripheral pulse deficit, murmurs and signs of heart failure. The spectrum of arrhythmias that may cause dizziness encompasses a wide variety of bradycardias and tachycardias (Table 4.18). Rarely, arrhythmia can be provoked by head turns of pressure applied to the neck due to a hypersensitive carotid sinus.

Pathophysiology

Brain perfusion suffers when heart rate falls below around 40/min or exceeds around 170/ min. Individual arrhythmia tolerance, however, varies considerably depending on concurrent factors such as ventricular filling and contractility, peripheral vascular tone and cerebral autoregulation. When asystole causes total cessation of cerebral blood flow, dizziness and other presyncopal symptoms start after three or four seconds and consciousness is lost after about ten seconds.

Investigations

Several arrhythmic disorders can be readily identified on routine ECG; examples are atrioventricular block, Wolff–Parkinson–White syndrome, atrial flutter and fibrillation. Paroxysmal arrhythmia, in contrast, usually requires Holter monitoring for 24 hours. For identification of symptomatic arrhythmia, patients have to document clinical events during

Table 4.18 Arrhythmia syndromes that may induce dizziness

Tachycardias
Sinus tachycardia
Atrial tachycardia
Atrial flutter/fibrillation
Atrioventricular tachycardia
Pre-excitation syndromes
Ventricular tachycardia
Bradycardias
Sick sinus syndrome Carotid sinus hypersensitivity
Atrioventricular block
Atrial fibrillation with bradyarrhythmia

the recording. Holter monitoring, however, is often disappointing with a yield of less than 10% in patients with suspected paroxysmal arrhythmia. Sensitivity can be increased with repeated monitoring. Selected patients with rare paroxysmal arrhythmia may profit from an implantable loop recorder which records cardiac rhythm continuously for many months. Cardiac stress testing on a treadmill is useful for detection of exercise-induced arrhythmia. Patients with potentially dangerous types of arrhythmia that cannot be reliably identified by non-invasive techniques may require intracardial electrophysiological testing. When carotid sinus hypersensitivity is suspected a causal relationship to the patient's dizziness should be established by recording an ECG during the individual provocative movement.

Differential diagnosis

Cardiac disorders other than arrhythmia may induce cerebral hypoperfusion leading to presyncope or syncope. Particular examples are congestive heart failure and valvular disease decreasing cardiac outflow, such as high-grade aortic stenosis. A characteristic feature of these disorders is symptom provocation by exertion due to redistribution of cardiac output from the cerebral circulation to the muscles. Orthostatic hypotension produces a similar type of dizziness but can be readily differentiated by the history (e.g. dizziness after standing up) and measurement of orthostatic blood pressure. Symptomatic arrhythmia can be difficult to differentiate from neurally mediated syncope or presyncope when there is no typical trigger pointing to a vascular reflex mechanism. In this situation, the following features should raise the suspicion of a cardiac arrhythmia: syncope or presyncope while supine, old age, known cardiac disease, abnormal resting ECG. Both extensive cardiological investigation and tilt-table testing may be necessary to settle doubtful cases.

Treatment

Correction of underlying disorders such as electrolyte or metabolic disturbances and elimination of arrhythmogenic drugs is the first line of therapy. Symptomatic treatment of arrhythmias includes antiarrhythmic drugs, cardiac pacemakers, implantable cardioverter defibrillators and radio-frequency catheter ablation of arrhythmogenic structures within the heart. The role of antiarrhythmic drugs has decreased considerably since a large placebo-controlled study has shown that antiarrhythmic drugs may in fact increase mortality due to arrhythmia.

Panic attacks

Table 4.19 Panic attacks: key features

History	Attacks with intense fear and associated somatic symptoms; may coexist with vestibular disorder
Clinical findings	Normal with pure panic attacks, but abnormalities from subclinical vestibular dysfunction or vestibular disease not uncommon
Pathophysiology	Often related to anxiety disorders, increased attention to body signals and conditioned responses; sometimes triggered by experience of vestibular dysfunction Additional hyperventilation may cause dizziness from cerebral hypoperfusion
Investigations	Vestibular testing, psychiatric opinion
Treatment	Cognitive behavioural therapy, sometimes vestibular rehabilitation or anxiolytic/antidepressant medication

Dizziness of psychological origin may occur acutely as a symptom of panic attacks or chronically in the form of persistent perceptual dizziness (see Chapter 6).

Clinical features

Panic attacks are defined as periods of intense anxiety or discomfort with at least four of the symptoms listed in Table 4.20. Dizziness occurs in more than half of patients with panic attacks. When there are fewer than four symptoms altogether the term 'limited-symptom attacks' is used, which is not uncommon in patients presenting with a main complaint of dizziness. Many attacks start 'out of the blue' but they can be triggered by body sensations, such as an accelerated heartbeat after a cup of coffee. The onset of an attack is rapid and duration is mostly in the order of 10–20 minutes; occasional attacks may last more than an hour.

Panic attacks often start in early adulthood and affect women more often than men. There is a genetic predisposition, but the first manifestation is commonly during a period of stressful life events such as a new job, death of a family member or an acute cardiac or vestibular illness. They are maintained by mistaken beliefs ('these symptoms must be dangerous') and negative/anxious self-talk ('what if I fall down and nobody helps me?').

Panic disorder is characterised by recurrent panic attacks and a persistent fear of having future panic attacks. This may lead to avoidance of situations in which attacks have occurred previously or which would be difficult to handle in case of another attack. Typical situations include going to movies or theatres, public transport, escalators, supermarkets, crowds or wide places. Phobic avoidance of these situations is called *agoraphobia*, which may eventually restrict patients to their homes as the only place where they feel safe.

Dizziness related to panic attacks is described by patients as light-headedness, feeling 'spaced out', wobbliness, shakiness, fear of falling, impending faint or a rocking or spinning sensation, sometimes even with spinning of the environment. For discrimination from a

Table 4.20 Symptoms of panic attacks

Palpitations or accelerated heart rate
Sweating
Trembling or shaking
Sensations of shortness of breath or smothering
Feeling of choking
Chest pain or discomfort
Nausea or abdominal distress
Feeling dizzy, unsteady, light-headed or faint
Derealisation (feelings of unreality) or depersonalisation (being detached from oneself)
Fear of losing control or going insane
Sense of impending death
Paraesthesias
Chills or hot flushes

vestibular type of vertigo it is useful to ask whether nausea and vomiting have occurred, whether the patient has actually fallen, whether bystanders have noticed any imbalance or veering to one side, and whether the patient has experienced true oscillopsia with constant movement of the environment in one direction as would be expected from a spontaneous vestibular nystagmus. However, an unusual type of the dizziness itself is certainly not sufficient to identify its psychological origin. Instead, positive evidence has to be elicited such as dizziness in the context of panic attacks, catastrophic cognitions, which are disproportionate for the actual events, and avoidance behaviour. In addition, clinical and laboratory findings should be either negative or unable to explain the current disability. An example would be a unilateral caloric hyporesponsiveness from an old vestibular neuritis in a patient who cannot leave his house because of attacks with dizziness and panic.

Evidence of both psychological and somatic elements is not uncommon in dizzy patients. Several studies have shown that patients with panic disorder frequently have abnormalities on vestibular tests. A common clinical pattern is anxiety-related dizziness evolving from a well-defined vestibular syndrome such as benign positional vertigo or vestibular neuritis. This may lead to severe persisting disability, which may last for years after the initial vertigo has resolved.

Vice versa, panic attacks may be complicated by somatic dizziness when a patient starts to hyperventilate. Instead of enquiring directly about hyperventilation (which often yields a 'no') one can ask: 'Have you felt short of breath?' or 'Have you noticed a dry mouth?' Numbness around the mouth and in the fingers is frequently associated, while tonic contractions of lip, hand and feet muscles ensues only from prolonged overbreathing.

Pathophysiology

Panic attacks are commonly triggered and maintained by an interaction of catastrophic thoughts and unpleasant body sensations, and either of the two may come first. This establishes a vicious circle of anxious cognition producing somatic reactions such as sweating, trembling and palpitations, which in turn are misinterpreted as signalling imminent danger leading to even more anxiety. The mechanism of conditioning decreases the threshold for further attacks and eventually produces dramatic responses to completely harmless stimuli such as spontaneous variations of heartbeat.

In patients with anxiety-related dizziness following a vestibular disorder, the initial somatic symptoms represent an unconditioned aversive stimulus provoking anxiety. So-called 'interoceptive conditioning' may then lead to panic attacks in response to mild vestibular symptoms or physiological vestibular sensations. Since vestibular symptoms tend to be aggravated by specific situations, agoraphobia may develop as a learned avoidance behaviour. Cognitive mechanisms may contribute to this process, when vestibular symptoms are interpreted catastrophically, thus inducing panic attacks.

Hyperventilation-induced dizziness is caused by cerebral vasoconstriction and consecutive global hypoperfusion affecting predominantly the cerebral cortex with its high oxygen demand.

Investigations

In patients with panic attacks, thyroid hormone levels and TSH should be obtained to rule out hyperthyroidism. Vestibular testing including caloric responses is useful for detection of vestibular dysfunction, although subclinical abnormalities that are not reflected by the patient's history and clinical findings usually play a contributory rather than causative role in patients with disabling dizziness. Psychiatric assessment is advisable for establishing a firm diagnosis and for selection of appropriate treatment measures.

Symptom provocation by forceful voluntary hyperventilation for up to three minutes is sometimes used as a test for hyperventilation-induced dizziness. The weakness of the hyperventilation test is its low specificity as any normal person gets dizzy and unsteady when hyperventilating long enough. The specificity increases when patients recognise their typical dizziness and associated symptoms during the test. Simultaneous observation of the eyes with Frenzel's glasses may serve to identify a hyperventilation-induced nystagmus pointing to an underlying vestibular disorder, particularly acoustic neuroma (see page 90).

Differential diagnosis

Panic attacks secondary to an underlying cause may occur with hyperthyroidism, pheo-chromocytoma, hypoglycaemia, use of caffeine, marijuana, cocaine, amphetamine and also during withdrawal of alcohol, benzodiazepines or SSRI (selective serotonine reuptake inhibitors) antidepressants. When a patient reports a different type of dizziness or vertigo occurring between attacks, further enquiry and investigations are necessary to identify other treatable conditions such as poorly compensated unilateral vestibular loss or vestibular migraine. Sometimes, dizziness due to panic attacks must be distinguished from neurally mediated presyncope triggered by an emotional stimulus such as the sight of blood, but the associated symptoms of either panic attacks (see Table 4.20) or presyncope (dimming of vision, ringing in the ears, subsequent syncope) will usually point to the correct diagnosis. Very rarely, intense anxiety and dizziness are the leading symptoms of focal epileptic seizures from the temporal lobe (see page 90).

Treatment

A diagnosis of panic attacks should be discussed with the patient as frankly as one would do with any other disease. Most patients open up when psychological symptoms are regarded as real and as serious as somatic ones, when psychological issues are addressed with empathy, and when the mechanisms by which thoughts and emotions may induce somatic symptoms are well explained.

Numerous studies have shown the efficacy of cognitive behavioural therapy (CBT) for treating panic attacks with or without agoraphobia. This approach combines desensitisation by graded exposure to anxiety-inducing stimuli with cognitive therapy which aims to redefine what the patient thinks about anxiety-provoking situations, symptoms and his/her own coping strategies (Figure 4.4). Vestibular rehabilitation shares several features with CBT, such as deliberate exposure to the symptom-provoking situation and professional advice while experiencing the symptoms (see Chapter 8). Vestibular rehabilitation can therefore be a suitable addition or the sole treatment for patients who do not wish to undergo psychotherapy.

Drug-induced dizziness

Medication side-effects rank among the most common causes of dizziness but rarely cause a patient to see a neurologist or ENT specialist. Usually, onset of the problem after

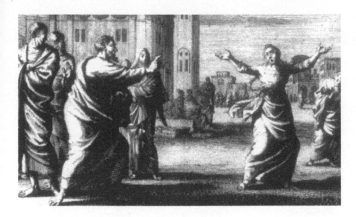

Figure 4.4 Obsession or agoraphobia with panic attacks? In the Middle Ages, psychiatric disease was explained by demonic obsession and treated with exorcism. Today, the figure may serve to illustrate healing from agoraphobia by in-vivo desensitisation: an agoraphobic patient is taken to the market place by her behavioural therapist. (From: Charcot JM, Richer P, *Die Besessenen in der Kunst* (German reissue). Göttingen: Steidl 1988, with permission.)

prescription of a new drug, or with incremental doses as well as the associated side-effects, makes the cause of dizziness obvious to the patient and the treating doctor. An exception to this rule is bilateral vestibular loss due to ototoxicity which may be diagnosed only years after the patient has developed balance problems. Drug-induced dizziness can be episodic or fluctuating when plasma concentrations vary according to dosing intervals and the pharmacokinetics of the drug. On the other hand, dizziness may be persistent when high plasma concentrations are maintained and even permanent when brain or inner-ear structures are damaged. This chapter, although principally dedicated to *recurrent* dizziness, will deal with all these types of drug-induced dizziness. Our classification of drugs is oriented towards their pathophysiologic mechanisms causing: sedation, vestibular suppression, ototoxicity, cerebellar toxicity, peripheral neuropathy, orthostatic hypotension, hypoglycaemia, and 'unknown' (Table 4.21).

Sedation

Benzodiazepines and other sedating drugs are a major risk factor for falls and hip fractures in the elderly. These drugs cause dizziness and unsteadiness for various reasons. Drowsiness and poor concentration interfere with spatial orientation at the cortical level; concomitant vestibular suppression reduces processing of signals within the labyrinth and the vestibular nuclei; and slowed reaction times impair postural adjustments during unexpected challenges of balance, thus promoting falls. At higher doses this may be complemented by cerebellar toxicity.

Vestibular suppression

It seems paradoxical, but antivertiginous medication can make you dizzy! These drugs suppress the vestibular system indiscriminately, acting on both erroneous signals resulting from vestibular disorders and useful information as required for spatial orientation, vestibulo-ocular reflexes and balance. Since central compensation after unilateral vestibular loss depends on normal input from the intact side and restoration of nuclear activity on the affected side, this class of drugs may impair recovery when given for more than just a day or two. In addition, vestibular suppression is difficult to obtain without sedation which itself may cause dizziness. Therefore, it is recommended to use vestibular suppressants essentially for short-term treatment of patients with acute vestibular disease or motion sickness (see page 175).

Table 4.21 Drugs causing dizziness and imbalance

Mechanism	Class of drugs	Sample drug
Sedation	Benzodiazepines	Diazepam, alprazolam, lorazepam
	Other GABAergic substances	Gabapentin, pregabalin
	Barbiturates	Phenobarbitone
	Aliphatic phenothiazines	Chlorpromazine
	Opiates	Morphine, codeine
Vestibular suppression	Antihistamines	Dimenhydrinate, promethazine
	Benzodiazepines	Diazepam, lorazepam
	Anticholinergics	Scopolamine
Ototoxicity	Aminoglycosides	Gentamicin, streptomycin
	Glycopeptide antibiotics	Vancomycin
	Alkylating agents	Cisplatin
	Loop diuretics (reversible)	Furosemide, ethacrynic acid
	NSAIDS (reversible)	Aspirin, ibuprofen
	Antimalarial drugs (reversible)	Quinine, quinidine
Cerebellar toxicity	Antiepileptics	Carbamazepine, phenytoin, phenobarbitone, gabapentine, lamotrigine
	Benzodiazepines	Diazepam, clonazepam
	Inorganic salt	Lithium salt
	Other GABAergic substances	Gabapentin, pregabalin
	Antimetabolites	Cytarabine
	Antiarrhythmics	Amiodarone
Peripheral neuropathy	Chemotherapeutics	Vincristine, paclitaxel, cisplatin, bortezomib
	Antiretrovirals	Stavudine, didanosine, zalcitabine
	Tuberculostatics	Isoniazid
	Antiarrhythmics	Amiodarone
Orthostatic hypotension	Diuretics	Thiazide diuretics, furosemide
	Vasodilators	Nitroglycerine, isosorbide
	Beta-blockers	Propranolol, metoprolol
	Alpha-blockers	Phenoxybenzamine, prazosin
	Calcium-channel blockers	Nifedipine
	ACE inhibitors	Captopril, enalapril
	AT1-receptor antagonists	Losartan, candesartan
	Tricyclic antidepressants	Amitryptyline
	Aliphatic phenothiazines	Clorpromazine
	Dopaminergics	L-dopa, pergolide
	MAO inhibitors	Tranylcypromine
Hypoglycaemia	Antidiabetics	Insulin, Sulfonylurea
	Beta-blockers	Propranolol
	MAO inhibitors	Tranylcypromine
Unknown	Antimalarial	Mefloquin
	Antibiotics	Ofloxazin, trovafloxacin, minocycline
	And many more . . .	

ACE = angiotensin-converting enzyme; MAO = monoamine oxidase

Ototoxicity

Aminoglycoside antibiotics such as gentamicin and other drugs may cause irreversible damage to the vestibular sensory epithelia, particularly when applied to a patient with renal failure. The resulting bilateral loss of vestibular function causes oscillopsia during head motion and imbalance which worsens in darkness (see page 141). The typical patient with aminoglycoside ototoxicity reports that symptoms started after he or she was in an intensive care unit for cardiac surgery or sepsis. Note that gentamicin, the most common ototoxic drug, has only minor effects on hearing, so patients do not report serious deafness. Nowadays, many Gram-negative infections can be managed without aminoglycoside antibiotics, which holds the promise that the number of patients with iatrogenic irreversible loss of vestibular function may decrease in the future.

Cerebellar toxicity

When dizziness and imbalance are related to ataxia and the Romberg test is negative (i.e. unsteadiness is present with eyes open and does not increase substantially after eye closure), cerebellar dysfunction is very likely. Drug-induced cerebellar toxicity is characterised by a subacute onset and bilateral involvement with gaze-evoked nystagmus as an early feature, later followed by downbeat nystagmus, limb ataxia and dysarthria. The most common offending drugs are lithium, tranquillisers and antiepileptics such as phenytoin, carbamazepine and lamotrigin, and the antineoplastic agent cytarabine. Rarely, cerebellar dysfunction may persist after the drug has been discontinued, particularly after lithium, phenytoin and cytarabine intoxication.

Peripheral neuropathy

Peripheral neuropathy causes somatosensory de-afferentation leading to unsteadiness and spatial disorientation which patients report as dizziness (see page 153). Several chemotherapeutic agents are most aggressive in this respect causing rapidly progressive, irreversible damage to the peripheral nerves. The only chance for an affected patient is rapid recognition of the problem by an observant doctor and termination of the drug.

Orthostatic hypotension

A drop of blood pressure immediately after standing up is called 'orthostatic hypotension' (see page 94). Drugs are a common causative or contributory factor, particularly antihypertensives in elderly patients. Therefore, measuring the resting supine or seated blood pressure only may be insufficient to monitor treatment in these patients.

Hypoglycaemia

While spontaneous hypoglycaemia is rare, many diabetic patients experience hypoglycaemia due to insulin or oral antidiabetics. Dizziness seldom occurs in isolation but rather as part of the hypoglycaemic symptom cluster which includes hunger, perspiration, shakiness, poor concentration, irritability, mood swings, feeling anxious or weak, confusion, abnormal behaviour, somnolence and ultimately coma. The diagnosis is confirmed when the blood sugar level is below 70 mg/dL during symptomatic episodes and when glucose administration leads to rapid resolution of symptoms.

Unknown

About one-quarter of licensed drugs have been reported to cause dizziness as an adverse effect, but often the mechanism is unclear.

Other causes of recurrent dizziness

Hypertension

*Hyper*tension is often held to be a common cause of dizziness, but quite wrongly so. Cerebral autoregulation protects the brain from the effects of systemic hypertension. However, dizziness can be a symptom of *hypertensive crisis*, a condition affecting about 1% of hypertensive individuals at some time which ensues when *diastolic* blood pressure is maintained above 120 mmHg. Associated symptoms and signs may include headache, visual blurring, confusion, lethargy, retinal haemorrhages and exudates, papilloedema, focal neurological signs and seizures. MRI may show white-matter oedema, predominantly affecting the occipital and parietal lobes, so-called posterior reversible encephalopathy syndrome (PRES). Dizziness and other neurological symptoms are caused by cerebral hypoperfusion due to arteriolar spasm and cerebral oedema.

Metabolic disorders and general medical conditions

Disorders such as uraemia, hepatic failure, hypoglycaemia, electrolyte imbalance or thyrotoxicosis may present with dizziness, but usually there are other more typical features indicating metabolic encephalopathy, including confusion, agitation, sleepiness, trembling and negative myoclonus (asterixis). Also consider anaemia in a patient with chronic dizziness and fatigue.

Height vertigo

This is, strictly speaking, a misnomer because affected individuals feel dizzy and unstable rather than vertiginous when they are exposed to heights. A typical provocative situation would be looking down from a roof or a cliff. Height vertigo has a physiological and a psychological dimension. The physiological aspect is that in opened-up places there is no visual environment at short distance which is normally needed to detect body sway visually. Thus, balance control is restricted to somatosensory and vestibular input. This corresponds to an eyes-closed situation which would normally decrease postural stability somewhat but should not cause any dizziness or imbalance. But imagine standing with eyes closed next to an unprotected cliff and you will understand the psychological side of the problem. It is the *potential* danger and the imagination of falling which makes one feel uncomfortable and some people even 'frightened to death'. When height vertigo, which most of us have experienced to some degree, becomes height phobia, treatment with behavioural therapy may be required. In less complicated cases it may be sufficient to step back or hold on to a support in order to provide somatosensory substitution for the lack of visual information.

What to do if you don't have a clue

As with recurrent vertigo, the cause of recurrent dizziness may remain obscure even after thorough investigation. In the following we have listed some questions and reminders that may increase the diagnostic yield.

Is it really dizziness?

Remember that verbal representation of a symptom is not the symptom itself and that most patients have difficulty in expressing what they have experienced. In addition, mild forms of vertigo often do not have the typical spinning quality, partly because visual fixation can suppress peripheral vestibular nystagmus. Questioning about previous spinning sensations, positional provocation, oscillopsia, nausea and veering to one side may point to vestibular vertigo rather than non-vestibular dizziness. Vestibular testing may reveal a labyrinthine disorder. Nevertheless, one should not overinterpret isolated minor abnormalities and borderline pathological findings on vestibular testing because they are common in healthy people. Patients with unsteadiness and disequilibrium may likewise complain about recurrent dizziness. Dizziness in these patients occurs exclusively during standing and walking, and abnormal posture or gait should be visible on inspection or neurological examination (Table 6.2, page 133).

Have you missed a relevant detail from the history?

A meticulous history may be necessary to identify previous somatic and psychiatric disorders, precipitating factors, associated symptoms or offending drugs. A dizziness diary is often helpful to record symptoms accurately and to document the temporal profile of episodic complaints.

Don't use 'psychogenic dizziness' as a waste basket for undiagnosed patients

Nowadays, psychiatric diagnoses are based on operational criteria as defined by DSM-5 or ICD-11. A false diagnosis, no matter if psychogenic or somatic, is detrimental for the patient with regard to appropriate treatment and coping. When psychological factors appear to be involved it is useful to obtain psychiatric consultation *and* to pursue the appropriate somatic investigations before weighing the contributions of each to the problem.

Ask for consultation in internal medicine

As a neurologist or ENT specialist you will usually refer dizzy patients to internal medicine after the search for a vestibular or neurological disorder has been negative. Again, any abnormal finding should be critically evaluated for its clinical relevance, to protect the patient from unnecessary measures such as a cardiac pacemaker for a vasodepressor type of neurally mediated syncope.

Positional vertigo

5

Positional vertigo occurs exclusively or predominantly with specific head positions (Table 5.1). Identification of positional vertigo is usually straightforward from the history: patients complain of vertigo that appears in certain head positions, such as after lying down or sitting up, after turning in bed from one side to the other, with head extension or bending forward. Occasionally, however, the positional nature of the vertigo is not recognised by the patient, even after questioning. Therefore, positional tests should be performed in all patients with recurrent vertigo.

Table 5.1 Positional vertigo: common diagnoses with key features

Disorder	Key features
Posterior canal BPPV*, > 80% of all positional vertigo (page 109)	Brief attacks (< 30 s), provoked by turning in bed, lying down, sitting up from lying, head extension or bending over Symptomatic episodes for weeks to months, remissions for years Mainly torsional nystagmus beating towards the ground in lateral head-hanging position
Horizontal canal BPPV, < 20% of all positional vertigo (page 117)	Attacks mainly provoked by turning in bed Head-lateral positions provoke transient horizontal nystagmus towards the ground (canalolithiasis) or persistent horizontal nystagmus away from the ground (cupulolithiasis)
Anterior canal BPPV (page 123)	Attacks mainly provoked by lying down and sitting up. Nystagmus beats vertically downward, with minor torsional component towards the affected ear
Vestibular migraine (page 123)	May present with predominant positional vertigo History of migraine Migraine features during vertigo Symptomatic episodes from minutes to days Persistent positional nystagmus in any direction
Central positional vertigo (page 124)	Variable duration of single attacks, variable provoking positions and nystagmus features

Table 5.1 (*cont.*)

Disorder	Key features
	Additional brainstem or cerebellar signs possible
	May mimic single features of BPPV, but not the whole syndrome
Other causes (page 127)	Positional alcohol vertigo and nystagmus, perilymph fistula, vestibular paroxysmia, macroglobulinaemia, amiodarone toxicity, head-extension vertigo

* BPPV = benign paroxysmal positional vertigo

Some authors distinguish between *positional* and *positioning vertigo*. The former term implies that vertigo continues as long as the head is kept in the provocative position, whereas the latter term is used for vertigo that subsides while the head remains in the critical position. This nomenclature has not been widely accepted, probably because it does not reliably separate peripheral from central vestibular disorders.

Posterior canal benign paroxysmal positional vertigo

Table 5.2 Posterior canal benign paroxysmal positional vertigo: key features

History	Brief attacks of vertigo (< 30 s), provoked by turning in bed, lying down, sitting up from lying, head extension or bending over Symptomatic episodes for weeks to months, asymptomatic intervals for months to years
Clinical findings	Hallpike positional testing: mainly torsional nystagmus, fast-phase directed towards the ground (+ smaller upward component) when positioned on the symptomatic side Often reversal nystagmus after sitting up
Pathophysiology	Dislodged otoconia from the utricle moving within the posterior canal after changes of head position
Investigations	Not required in typical cases
Treatment	Epley's or Semont's manoeuvre; modified Epley's for self-treatment at home

Clinical features

Benign paroxysmal positional vertigo (BPPV) is by far the most common cause of positional vertigo, accounting for about 80% of patients. Moreover, BPPV is the number one vestibular disorder, causing about 25% of referrals to specialised dizziness clinics. The prevalence of BPPV increases with advancing age, reaching at least 10% in the population over 80 years. Women are affected almost twice as often as men. BPPV may involve each semicircular canal, with BPPV of the posterior canal being the most common variant. All subtypes of BPPV can be diagnosed on the basis of clinical observation. The revelation of its pathophysiology has made BPPV the most successfully treatable cause of vertigo.

Benign paroxysmal positional vertigo of the posterior canal (PC-BPPV) causes brief attacks of vertigo which are precipitated by changes of head position. Patients typically experience vertigo when they turn over in bed, lie down from sitting, sit up from lying, extend the neck to look up, or bend over. The illusion of movement is usually rotatory, but a sensation of body tilt can also occur. Other complaints during the attack include imbalance, oscillopsia and occasionally nausea and vomiting. Patients are usually aware that certain head movements precipitate attacks of vertigo. They often develop strategies to avoid vertiginous attacks, such as lying down slowly, sleeping propped up or holding their neck stiff, which may lead to immobility and prolongation of the natural course of the disease. A secondary anxiety disorder with or without dizziness may persist even after BPPV has resolved.

A single attack of PC-BPPV usually lasts 5–20 seconds and hardly any longer than half a minute. However, after a flurry of attacks, patients may complain of prolonged dizziness and imbalance lasting from hours to days. Typically, PC-BPPV manifests itself with symptomatic episodes lasting from a few days to several months, which are interspersed by asymptomatic intervals of several months' to years' duration. Most cases of BPPV are idiopathic, but about 25% develop after head trauma or on the background of a pre-existing labyrinthine disorder such as vestibular neuritis or Ménière's disease. Bilateral involvement is rare in idiopathic BPPV but not uncommon in post-traumatic patients.

The diagnosis is confirmed by provocation of vertigo by positional testing and observation of typical nystagmus with or without Frenzel's glasses. The classic test for provocation and confirmation of PC-BPPV is the Hallpike manoeuvre (Figure 5.1). With this procedure the affected posterior canal is rotated in a plane parallel to gravity which ensures its maximal stimulation. Alternatively, a lateral tilt of the trunk and head from a sitting position can be performed with the head turned 45 degrees to the *opposite* side, which positions the head with the lateral aspect of the occiput on to the couch. With both manoeuvres, the actual positioning of the posterior semicircular canal is identical (video clips 02.16 to 02.19).

The diagnosis of benign paroxysmal positional vertigo of the posterior canal can be reliably made when the positional nystagmus fulfils the following criteria:

- *Torsional-vertical nystagmus.* This appears when the patient is positioned to the symptomatic side. The most prominent direction of nystagmus is a torsional component, beating with the upper pole of the eyes towards the undermost ear (video clip 05.01). In addition, there is a smaller vertical-upbeat nystagmus component, most prominent on the uppermost eye. As nystagmus direction is influenced by direction of gaze, the patient should fixate on the doctor's nose to keep the eyes close to primary gaze.
- *Latency.* Typically, nystagmus and vertigo start a few seconds after the precipitating head position is reached. Nystagmus intensity increases rapidly and then decays (crescendo–decrescendo).
- *Duration.* Nystagmus usually lasts 5–20 seconds and only rarely exceeds 30 seconds.

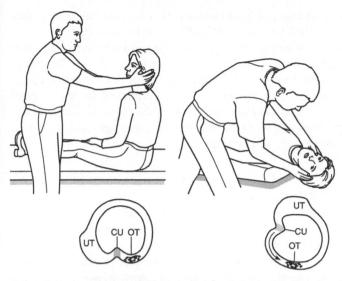

Figure 5.1 Hallpike positioning for identification of canalolithiasis of the left posterior canal. The man-oeuvre starts with the patient sitting upright on an examination couch with his head turned 45 degrees towards the examiner. She is instructed to keep her eyes open and to watch the examiner's forehead. Then the patient is swiftly moved to a lateral head-hanging position. The appearance of a transient, torsional-upward nystagmus indicates PC-BPPV of the lowermost ear. The mechanism of canalolithiasis is depicted in the lower part of the figure. When the patient is upright, otoconia are located at the base of the cupula and do not have any effect. During the Hallpike test, the head is rotated backwards in the plane of the posterior canal, inducing movement of the particles within the canal which leads to an endolymph and cupular displacement in the same direction. The ensuing activation of the canal's hair cells results in a mixed torsional-upward nystagmus which reflects the excitatory connections of the posterior canal with the superior oblique and the inferior rectus muscle. The nystagmus subsides after the particles have reached the most dependent point of the canal and the cupula has returned to the resting position. When the patient sits up again the particles will be shifted in the opposite direction causing inhibitory deflection of the cupula and hair cells, resulting in a reversed nystagmus. CU = Cupula, OT = Otoconia, UT = Utricle. (From: von Brevern M, Lempert T. Benigner paroxsymaler Lagerungsschwindel. *Nervenarzt* 2004; **75**: 1027–36, with permission.)

Video 05.01 – Right-sided posterior canal BPPV
The patient is being filmed after having attained the right-ear-down position with the Hallpike manoeuvre. A torsional right-beating nystagmus (anticlockwise nystagmus from the observer's point of view) is shown and gradually disappears. This nystagmus is typical for right-sided posterior canal BPPV.

- *Reversal.* A few seconds after the patient has returned to the sitting position, a transient nystagmus of lesser intensity, which beats in the opposite direction, can be observed.
- *Fatigability.* Vertigo and nystagmus decrease with repeated positioning in most cases. However, repeated testing is distressing for the patient and is usually not required.

Unilateral PC-BPPV may mimic bilateral BPPV when during positional testing of the unaffected ear the head is rotated more than 45 degrees to the side, which stimulates the posterior canal of the opposite (symptomatic) ear.

Pathophysiology

Benign paroxysmal positional vertigo is caused by dislodged otoconia from the utricle, which may aggregate to a clot. When the clot has entered a semicircular canal, it causes inadequate endolymph flow after changes of head position. This concept has been termed *canalolithiasis* (Figure 5.1). All clinical features of PC-BPPV can be explained by canolo-lithiasis. Latency is probably caused by movement of the particles within the ampulla (before reaching the narrow duct) where they have only minor hydrodynamic effects. The limited duration of the nystagmus reflects the journey of the particles along the duct before they settle in its lowermost part. Nystagmus reversal after sitting up is explained by the reversed direction of particle migration leading to a cupular deflection in the opposite direction.

There are several factors predisposing to BPPV, namely advanced age, head trauma, a preceding inner-ear disease, osteoporosis and intubation for general surgery, which all fit the canalolithiasis concept of BPPV.

- *Age.* The number of otoconia attached to the utricle and sacculus decreases with age, possibly due to spontaneous dislodgement.
- *Trauma.* Even mild head trauma may loosen otoconia from the gelatinous surface of the utricular macula, leading to BPPV as soon as these particles have entered a semicircular canal, which usually occurs within a few days.
- *Inner-ear disease.* Vestibular neuritis or other peripheral vestibular disease may cause BPPV by damaging the utricle, resulting in a coexistence of caloric hyporesponsiveness and BPPV. This seemingly paradoxical finding is explained by the posterior canal being spared, which is common in vestibular neuritis and may also occur in other inner-ear disorders.
- *Osteoporosis.* Impaired calcium metabolism leads to abnormal otolith formulation which may easily dissolve from the macula.
- *Surgery.* BPPV frequently manifests itself in the postoperative phase of all types of surgery, which may be explained by head reclination for intubation during general anaesthesia, allowing the mobile otoconia to enter the posterior canal.

Migraine is another established risk factor, but the mechanism which links the two disorders is unknown.

The canalolithiasis concept is supported by several histological and intra-operative findings. Schuknecht described granular deposits both on the cupula and within the semicircular canal in patients who suffered from PC-BPPV prior to death from unrelated disease. Mobile endolymph particles have been observed intra-operatively within the posterior canal in patients with BPPV (Figure 5.2). Recovered particles have proved morphologically consistent with degenerated otoconia when studied by electron microscopy. However, the most convincing proof for canalolithiasis comes from the efficacy of positioning manoeuvres, which clear the affected canal of mobile particles.

Investigations

In a patient with typical presentation no additional testing is required. Frenzel's glasses or video-oculography during positional testing can enhance nystagmus observation. A history of non-positional vertigo may point to an underlying labyrinthine disorder, which should be evaluated with vestibular and audiometric testing.

Differential diagnosis

Posterior canal benign paroxysmal positional vertigo must be differentiated from other forms of BPPV and from central positional vertigo due to a lesion of the vestibular nuclei or

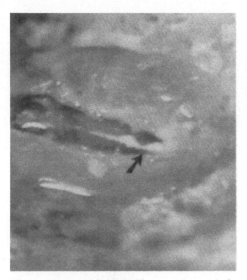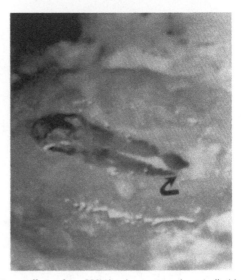

Figure 5.2 Canalolithiasis. The posterior canal of a patient suffering from BPPV has been opened surgically (dark area in the centre) showing white material within the endolymph which moves when the patient's head is raised (arrows). (From: Parnes, McClure 1992, with permission.)

Table 5.3 Differential diagnosis of positional nystagmus

Disorder	Latency	Duration	Direction
Posterior canal BPPV	Yes	5–30 s	Torsional towards lower ear with vertical upward component; reversal after sitting up common
Horizontal canal BPPV, canalolithiasis	No	10–60 s	Horizontal to the ground in either head-lateral position
Horizontal canal BPPV, cupulolithiasis	Often	> 2 min	Horizontal away from the ground in either head-lateral position
Anterior canal BPPV, canalolithiasis	Possible	< 1 min	Downbeat and torsional; fast phases of torsion pointing to the affected side (torsion often not visible)
Central positional vertigo	Usually no latency	Usually persistent	Often pure upbeat/downbeat; any combination of provoking position and nystagmus direction possible
Positional vertigo due to vestibular migraine	Usually no latency	Persistent	Any combination of provoking position and nystagmus direction possible

caudal cerebellum. The distinction is mainly based on nystagmus features (Table 5.3). A history of recurrences and remissions over years is a strong argument in favour of BPPV and against a central lesion. Differentiation from vestibular migraine (see page 124) and central positional vertigo (page 125) is discussed below.

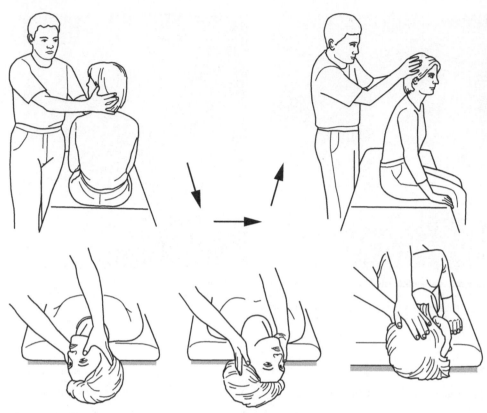

Figure 5.3 **Epley's canalith repositioning procedure for treatment of PC-BPPV on the left.** The procedure consists of a set of five successive head positionings that are hand-guided by a therapist. Each positioning is performed rapidly and is maintained for 30 seconds. From left to right: sit patient upright with head turned 45 degrees to affected side. Lie patient down with head dependent as if performing Dix–Hallpike manoeuvre. Rotate head through 90 degrees to opposite side with face upwards, maintaining dependent position. Rotate head and body further so that patient is facing obliquely downward, with nose 45 degrees below horizontal. Raise patient to a sitting position. (From: von Brevern M, Lempert T. Benigner paroxsymaler Lagerungsschwindel. *Nervenarzt* 2004; **75**: 1027–36, with permission.) See video clips 05.04 and 05.05.

Treatment

The first therapeutic step is informing the patient about the mechanism and benign course of BPPV, which relieves unnecessary fears and prepares the patient for the management of the disorder. There are two treatment procedures for PC-BPPV which induce the return of otolithic debris from the posterior canal back into the utricle where they no longer produce positional vertigo, namely Epley's and Semont's manoeuvres. These therapies are highly effective in terminating an acute episode of PC-BPPV, but they have no influence on future recurrences which can be expected in about half of the patients after several months or, more commonly, years.

- Epley introduced the canalith repositioning procedure, in which the posterior canal is rotated backwards close to its planar orientation (Figure 5.3, video clips 05.04 and 05.05). The manoeuvre consists of a series of successive head positionings each of

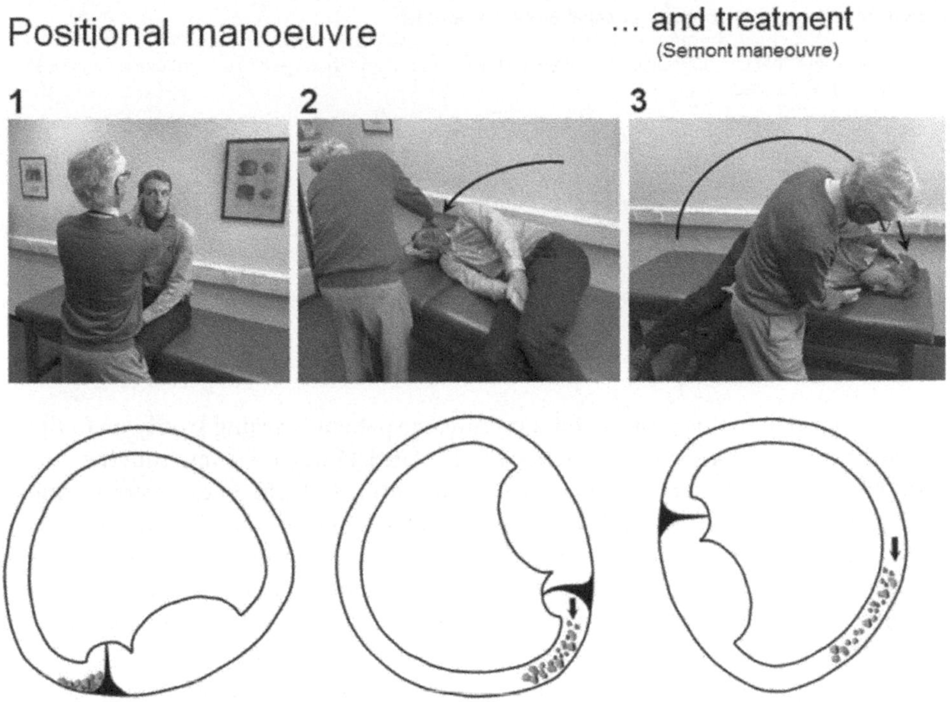

Positional manoeuvre

... and treatment
(Semont maneouvre)

1 **2** **3**

Figure 5.4 Semont's manoeuvre for treatment of PC- BPPV on the right. *Top:* the procedure is hand-guided by a therapist. All movements are performed rapidly. The head is turned 45 degrees away from the affected ear throughout the manoeuvre. From left to right: sit patient upright with head turned 45 degrees away from affected side. Lie patient down to affected side maintaining 45 degrees head rotation and wait for 1 minute. Swing head and body rapidly to the opposite side with the head still turned in the same direction. In the new position the nose is 45 degrees below horizontal. Wait for 1 minute. Raise patient to a sitting position. *Bottom:* movement of otoconia towards the utricle during the manoeuvre. See also video clips 05.02 and 05.03.

about 90 degrees, displacement. For observation of nystagmus, patients should be instructed to keep their eyes open. A positional nystagmus appearing in the second and third head position, which beats in the same direction with respect to the head, indicates successive movement of the particles towards the utricle and predicts a favourable outcome. A frequent cause of failure is insufficient head reclination during transition from one head-hanging position to the other, causing particles to move back towards the cupular end of the canal. Vibration of the mastoid during the procedure has been recommended but does not improve treatment outcome. Staying upright for 48 hours after successful treatment improves the outcome slightly, but has to be traded off against the imposed discomfort. Sleeping on the unaffected side may have a similar effect and seems more practical.

- The Semont manoeuvre involves a 180-degree swing of the head in the plane of the posterior canal (Figure 5.4, video clips 5.02 and 5.03). The examiner guides the manoeuvre by standing in front of the patient who is seated on a couch with the head rotated 45 degrees away from the affected ear. Then the patient is brought with a fast movement to a lying position on the side of the affected ear. In this position, vertigo is triggered with torsional nystagmus beating towards the affected (undermost) ear.

Video 05.02 – Treatment of posterior canal BPPV: Semont left
The patient is examined with the left ear down. From that position the patient is swung all the way from the left-ear-down position to the right eye position on the other end of the couch and then back to upright again. Each position is maintained for 30 seconds.

Video 05.03 – Treatment of posterior canal BPPV: Semont right
The patient is first examined for BPPV of the right ear with a sideways right-sided Hallpike manoeuvre. After the nystagmus disappears the patient is rapidly swung from the end of the couch helped by holding on to the examiners as shown. The swinging movement should be in one single action from the right-ear-down position to the left eye down position on the other end of the couch. In that position the subject should wait for 30 seconds or until all nystagmus disappears.

After being kept in this position for a minute, the patient is swung swiftly on to the opposite side of the couch with the head still rotated 45 degrees away from the affected ear. In more simple terms, the patient is brought from an ear-down position on the affected side to an eye-down position on the opposite side. The manoeuvre is usually effective when another bout of vertigo appears in this position with nystagmus beating towards the affected (now uppermost) ear. Treatment failure may result from insufficient head rotation to the side and from slow execution of the 180-degree swing.

Epley and Semont manoeuvres are highly effective when performed properly. After a single application complete recovery is achieved in 50–70% of patients. When positional vertigo and nystagmus are still provokable, the manoeuvre should be repeated immediately which increases the success rate to 80–90%. Randomised controlled trials have shown that either manoeuvre is clearly more effective than a sham procedure or no treatment. When the Epley manoeuvre fails, the Semont manoeuvre can be performed as an alternative, or vice versa. Nausea can be prevented by vestibular sedatives administered before performing a therapeutic manoeuvre. Occasionally, a 'successful' liberatory manoeuvre may transform PC-BPPV into another type of BPPV by accidentally shifting particles into another semi-circular canal. Then, the appropriate manoeuvre for the affected canal will quickly relieve the patient's and the doctor's disappointment.

When a patient does not respond immediately to Epley's or Semont's procedure or suffers from frequent recurrences, a modified Epley procedure can be used for self-treatment at home. With adequate performance most patients become asymptomatic within a few days. This manoeuvre is also useful for patients with a suggestive history of BPPV but negative Hallpike testing in the clinic. Patients can identify the involved ear by doing the first step of the manoeuvre which corresponds to a Hallpike positional test. If the transition from sitting to right ear down provokes vertigo, the right labyrinth is affected. Figure 5.5 shows the manoeuvre for left and right BPPV. Patients with frequent relapses should be advised to avoid lowering their head below horizontal to prevent re-entry of otoconia into the posterior canal.

Surgery of the posterior canal can be considered in those exceptionally rare patients with long-standing BPPV who have not responded to appropriate and repeated therapeutic positionings. Both plugging of the posterior semicircular canal by the transmastoid approach and transection of the posterior ampullary nerve by a middle-ear approach have proven effective for permanent relief from PC-BPPV.

Horizontal canal benign paroxysmal positional vertigo: canalolithiasis type

Table 5.4 Horizontal canal benign paroxysmal positional vertigo of the canalolithiasis type: key features

History	Brief attacks of vertigo (< 60 s), provoked by turning in bed Symptomatic episodes for days to weeks, usually alternating with other variants of BPPV
Clinical findings	Positional testing with lateral head turns from supine Horizontal nystagmus on either side, fast phase directed towards the ground Stronger nystagmus on the symptomatic side
Pathophysiology	Dislodged otoconia from the utricle moving within the horizontal canal after changes of head position
Investigations	None in typical cases
Treatment	270-degree barbecue roll (Epley's manoeuvre modified for horizontal canal) towards the healthy side; or sleeping on the unaffected side.

BPPV = benign paroxysmal positional vertigo

Clinical features

Involvement of the horizontal canal accounts for 10–20% of all patients presenting with benign paroxysmal positional vertigo. Two variants have been described, namely the more common canalolithiasis (HC-canalolithiasis) and the rarer cupulolithiasis of the horizontal canal (HC-cupulolithiasis). The horizontal canal variants are important to recognise since they have features that have formerly been attributed to positional vertigo of central origin.

In HC-canalolithiasis, attacks of vertigo are provoked by turning the head to either side in the supine or reclined position, whereas sitting up or lying down produces fewer symptoms. Horizontal head movements in the upright position are usually well tolerated. Symptomatic episodes during which attacks of vertigo are provokable tend to be shorter than with involvement of the posterior canal, lasting from days to a few weeks. Patients with HC-canalolithiasis are often severely nauseated. Episodes of HC-canalolithiasis often alternate with other variants of BPPV.

For diagnostic positional testing the patient lies on his/her back and the head is turned rapidly from the nose-up to either lateral position. The supine lateral head turn provokes transient horizontal nystagmus beating towards the ground, regardless of whether the head is turned to the right or left (geotropic nystagmus). The typical nystagmus starts with no or minimal latency, beats purely horizontally with respect to the head, lasts up to one minute, changes direction when the head is turned to the opposite side and shows no or minimal fatigue with repetitive provocative manoeuvres. When the provoking position is maintained, a less intense but longer-lasting nystagmus with reversed direction may appear. Often, the typical nystagmus is also elicited by conventional Hallpike testing. Eye movements can be easily observed without Frenzel's glasses. Several nystagmus features help to identify the affected side:

1. Nystagmus is always stronger with the head turned to the side of the affected horizontal canal (video clip 05.06).

Video 05.04 – Treatment of posterior canal BPPV: Epley left
The manoeuvre starts with a conventional left-ear-down Hallpike manoeuvre. The doctor positions himself behind the patient and helps her to rotate the reclined head from left to right. The patient is then asked to lie down sideways on the right side and the patient's head is rotated to the right to bring the nose to point down 45° below horizontal. Finally the doctor helps the patient to sit up. It is important to allow 30 seconds in each of these positions so that the intracanalicular crystals have a chance to move to the new position within the posterior canal.

Video 05.05 – Treatment of posterior canal BPPV: Epley right
The manoeuvre starts with a conventional right-ear-down Hallpike manoeuvre. The doctor positions himself behind the patient's head so he can rotate the reclined head from right to left. After 30 seconds' rest the patient is asked to lie down fully sideways on her left side and the patient's head is rotated from right to left so that the nose points down 45° below horizontal. After the appropriate 30 seconds' rest the subject sits up again.

2. On this side nystagmus reversal is more pronounced.
3. The change from sitting to supine may provoke a transient horizontal nystagmus to the healthy side, while bending forward usually induces nystagmus to the affected side.

Pathophysiology

Like PC-BPPV, the HC-canalolithiasis variant is caused by aggregated otoconia which have entered a semicircular canal. A head turn to the affected ear while supine induces movement of the clot and endolymph flow towards the cupula which is located in the anterior portion of the canal. The resulting excitation of the horizontal canal's hair cells results in transient horizontal nystagmus beating to the affected side, i.e. to the undermost ear. The direction of nystagmus reverses with a head turn to the other side when the clot is shifted in the opposite direction (Figure 5.6). Spontaneous remission after a few days is common in HC-canalolithiasis because particles may leave the horizontal canal easily during natural head movements. In contrast, the posterior canal is predisposed to become an otolith trap owing to its anatomical orientation with its closed end in the lowermost position.

Investigations and differential diagnosis

In a patient with typical presentation no additional testing is required. A similar nystagmus may occasionally be produced by a central vestibular lesion involving the vestibular nuclei or the caudal cerebellum. However, recurrent episodes of BPPV, normal neurological findings and a rapid response to treatment favour a diagnosis of HC-canalolithiasis. Other forms of positional nystagmus are shown in Table 5.3.

Treatment

Several manoeuvres can be used to free the horizontal semicircular canal from otoconia. With the so-called barbecue rotation the supine patient is rotated 270 degrees in steps of 90 degrees in the plane of the horizontal canal towards the healthy side (Figure 5.7, video clips 5.07 and 5.08). With this manoeuvre, positional vertigo resolves in about 70% after one treatment session. Alternatively, the patient can be advised to rest or sleep sideways with the healthy ear below for eight hours, which similarly provides relief from further attacks in about 70% of the patients. A simple and equally effective treatment is

A

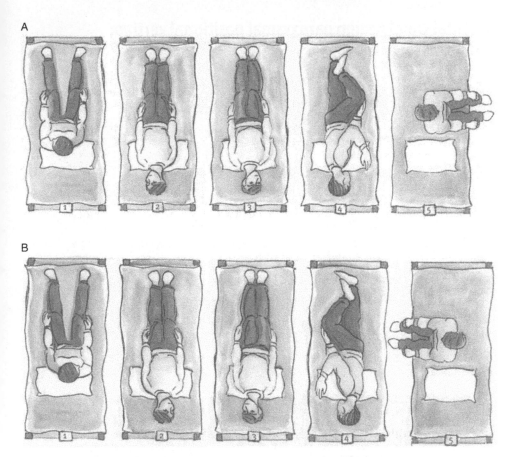

B

Figure 5.5 **A: Modified Epley's procedure for self-treatment of PC-BPPV on the left.** Instructions for the patient: (1) Start by sitting on a bed and turn your head 45 degrees to the left. Place a pillow behind you so that on lying back it will be under your shoulders. (2) Lie back quickly with shoulders on the pillow, neck extended, and head resting on the bed. In this position the affected (left) ear is underneath. Wait for 30 seconds. (3) Turn your head 90 degrees to the right without raising it and wait again for 30 seconds. (4) Turn your body and head another 90 degrees to the right and wait for another 30 seconds. (5) Sit up on the right side. This manoeuvre should be performed three times per day. Repeat this daily until you are free from positional vertigo for 24 hours. **B: Modified Epley's procedure for self-treatment of PC-BPPV on the right.** (1) Start by sitting on a bed and turn your head 45 degrees to the right. Place a pillow behind you so that on lying back it will be under your shoulders. (2) Lie back quickly with shoulders on the pillow, neck extended, and head resting on the bed. In this position the affected (right) ear is underneath. Wait for 30 seconds. (3) Turn your head 90 degrees to the left without raising it and wait again for 30 seconds. (4) Turn your body and head another 90 degrees to the left and wait for another 30 seconds. (5) Sit up on the left side. This manoeuvre should be performed three times per day. Repeat this daily until you are free from positional vertigo for 24 hours. (From: von Brevern M, Lempert T. Benigner paroxsymaler Lagerungsschwindel. *Nervenarzt* 2004; **75:** 1027–36, with permission.)

the Gufoni manoeuvre (video clips 05.09 and 05.10). The patient is brought quickly from a sitting position with the head turned 45° to the affected side into a side-lying position on the unaffected side where he remains for 1 minute. Then the head is turned 90 degrees towards the unaffected side (so that the nose points 45 degrees downwards) for 1 minute. Finally, the patient returns to sitting.

Horizontal canal benign paroxysmal positional vertigo: cupulolithiasis type

Table 5.5 Horizontal canal benign paroxysmal positional vertigo of the cupulolithiasis type: key features

History	Prolonged attacks of vertigo (> 3 min), provoked by turning in bed to the side Symptomatic episodes for days to weeks, usually alternating with other variants of BPPV
Clinical findings	Positional testing with head turns to the side from supine Horizontal nystagmus on either side, fast phase directed away from the ground Stronger nystagmus on the unaffected side
Pathophysiology	Dislodged otoconia from the utricle sticking to the cupula of the horizontal canal and causing cupular deflections in the head-lateral position
Investigations	None in typical cases
Treatment	Head percussion or shaking followed by 270-degree barbecue roll, towards the healthy side.

BPPV = benign paroxysmal positional vertigo

Video 05.06 – Canalolithiasis of the right horizontal canal
At the beginning of the video the supine patient turns her head 90 degrees to the left where a horizontal nystagmus to the left of moderate intensity can be observed. When the head is turned back to the nose-up position (after 27 s) the nystagmus disappears. When rotating the head to the right (after 42 s) a vigorous right-beating nystagmus sets in. This pattern of positional direction-changing nystagmus is called *geotropic* nystagmus because it beats toward the ground in either head-lateral position. In horizontal canalolithiasis the affected side corresponds to the one with the stronger nystagmus.

Video 05.07 – Barbecue manoeuvre for left horizontal BPPV
The treatment consists of a supine 270-degree head and body rotation in steps of 90 degrees. It starts from the nose-up position, then turning sequentially to the healthy (right) side, to the nose-down position and further to the left-ear-down position. Each position is held for 30 seconds. Finally, the patient sits up.

Video 05.08 – Barbecue manoeuvre for right horizontal BPPV
Treatment consists of a supine 270-degree head and body rotation in steps of 90 degrees. It starts from the nose-up position, then turning sequentially to the healthy (left) side, to the nose-down position and further to the right-ear-down position. Each position is held for 30 seconds. Finally, the patient sits up.

Clinical features

Patients with cupulolithiasis of the horizontal canal (HC-cupulolithiasis) suffer from positional vertigo mostly when they assume a lateral head position in bed. In contrast to HC-canalolithiasis, positional vertigo of HC-cupulolithiasis persists as long as the

Video 05.09 – Gufoni manoeuvre for left horizontal BPPV
The Gufoni manoeuvre starts from sitting. The patient is then positioned to the healthy (right) side. Note that we prefer to turn the head 45 degrees to the affected (left) side during this step (as opposed to the original description of the manoeuvre which proposed a straight head position with respect to the body). Thus, we want to make sure that the particles move towards the posterior (open) end of the canal. The next step is a head turn to a nose-down position (45 degrees to 60 degrees below horizontal). Each position is held for 30 seconds. Finally, the patient sits up.

Video 05.10 – Gufoni manoeuvre for right horizontal BPPV
The Gufoni manoeuvre starts from sitting. The patient is then positioned to the healthy (left) side. Note that we prefer to turn the head 45 degrees to the affected (right) side during this step (as opposed to the original description of the manoeuvre which proposed a straight head position with respect to the body). Thus, we want to make sure that the particles move towards the posterior (open) end of the canal. The next step is a head turn to a nose-down position (45 degrees to 60 degrees below horizontal). Each position is held for 30 seconds. Finally, the patient sits up.

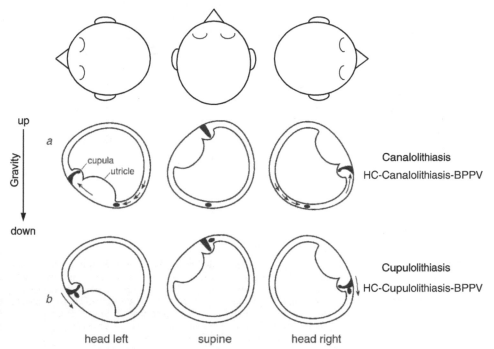

Figure 5.6 Mechanism of horizontal canalolithiasis and horizontal cupulolithiasis BPPV (right ear affected). In the canalolithiasis variant (**a**) the otoconial mass is moving freely within the canal, whereas in the cupulolithiasis variant (**b**) the mass is fixed to the cupula. In both conditions, deflections of the cupula reverse when the head is turned to the opposite lateral head position, explaining the direction-changing positional nystagmus. A critical difference between the two variants is the direction of cupular deflections, upward in canalolithiasis and downward in cupulolithiasis, which accounts for the geotropic nystagmus in canalolithiasis and the apogeotropic nystagmus in cupulolithiasis. Arrows indicate direction of cupular deflection

precipitating head-lateral position is held. HC-cupulolithiasis often alternates with other variants of BPPV and may especially develop during treatment of HC-canalolithiasis.

Typically, a head turn to either side in the supine position provokes long-lasting horizontal nystagmus beating away from the ground, a pattern which is called *apogeotropic nystagmus*. The nystagmus increases in intensity over 10–20 seconds and diminishes eventually but persists as long as the head is turned to the side. It is more intense with

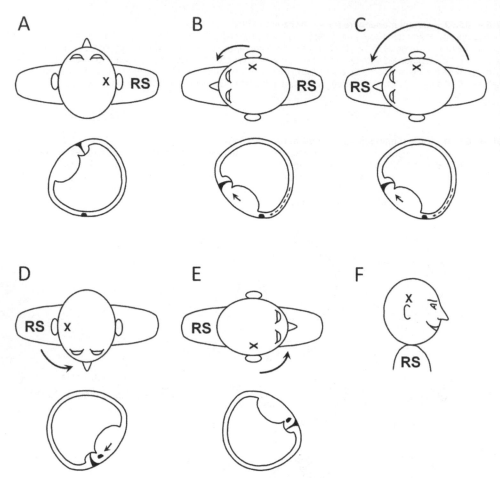

Figure 5.7 Barbecue rotation for treatment of horizontal canalolithiasis-BPPV on the right. *Top:* the supine patient is rotated 270 degrees in rapid steps of 90 degrees in the plane of the horizontal canal towards the healthy side. The time interval between each step is 30 seconds or until nystagmus has subsided. This positional manoeuvre can be used for self-treatment at home (with the head resting on the bed instead of being held by the examiner). From left to right: start in the supine nose-up position. Turn head 90 degrees to the left and rotate body by 180 degrees. Turn head to nose-down position. Turn head 90 degrees further to the left. Finally, sit patient up to his/her left side. *Bottom:* movement of otoconia towards the utricle during the manoeuvre.

the head turned to the healthy side. However, it may be missed when observed without Frenzel's glasses because of its slow build-up and its lower intensity as compared to the geotropic nystagmus of HC-canalolithiasis.

Pathophysiology

HC-cupulolithiasis is best explained with an otoconial mass sticking to the cupula thus making it sensitive to gravity. This concept explains both the apogeotropic nystagmus pattern (see Figure 5.6) and the long duration of nystagmus, which is due to the enduring deflection of the cupula in the provoking position. The slow persistent horizontal nystagmus in the supine position reflects the orientation of the cupula of the horizontal canal with respect to the head: when the patient lies with face up, gravity causes an excitatory deflection of the cupula, resulting in a nystagmus beating to the affected side.

Investigations and differential diagnosis

In a patient with typical presentation no additional testing is required. A similar nystagmus may be caused by a central vestibular lesion involving the vestibular nuclei or the caudal cerebellum. However, recurrent episodes of BPPV, normal neurological findings and a rapid response to treatment favour a diagnosis of HC-cupulolithiasis. Other forms of positional nystagmus are shown in Table 5.3.

Treatment

Only a few studies have evaluated the treatment of HC-cupulolithiasis. Gentle head percussion, vibration or fast head shakes of slow amplitude may dislodge otoconia from the cupula. As it is impossible to tell whether otoconia are sticking on the utricular or on the canal side of the cupula, this should be followed by a 270-degree barbecue roll or a Gufoni manoeuvre towards the healthy ear to force particles out of the canal (see Figure 5.7).

Video 05.11 – Cupulolithiasis of the right horizontal canal
Cupulolithiasis presents with long-lasting horizontal nystagmus in each head-lateral position beating away from the ground, i.e. towards the upper ear. This pattern of direction-changing positional nystagmus is called *apogeotropic* nystagmus. The affected side corresponds to the one with the weaker nystagmus which is the right side in this patient.

Anterior canal benign paroxysmal positional vertigo

The least common variant of BPPV affects the anterior canal (AC-BPPV). The rarity of AC-BPPV is probably related to its anatomical orientation which allows particles to leave the canal simply after lying down and sitting up again. AC-BPPV is provoked by Hallpike positioning, which stimulates particle migration within the affected anterior canal. Sometimes, the symptomatic side can be inferred from the nystagmus direction in the head-back or Hallpike position: it is always downbeat, but the torsional component is directed towards the affected ear. However, the torsional component may be too small for clinical observation, even when Frenzel's glasses are used. Given its rarity, the various positional treatment manoeuvres have not been validated. A more important concept is that the majority of positional downbeat nystagmuses are of central origin (e.g. midline cerebellar disorder) and hence most patients with positional downbeat nystagmus need to be imaged and assessed neurologically.

Vestibular migraine

Vestibular migraine is often aggravated by changes of head position and may present with pure positional vertigo for the duration of the acute attack. About half of the patients with vestibular migraine have experienced positional vertigo. Sometimes an episode of vestibular migraine starts with spontaneous vertigo, which becomes positional later on. Single bouts of vertigo may last a few seconds only or persist as long as the head position is maintained. Duration of symptomatic episodes during which positional nystagmus can be elicited varies from minutes to days. Recurrences are usually more frequent than in BPPV.

Positional nystagmus in vestibular migraine is usually persistent and corresponds to a central pattern with variable nystagmus directions, which are not systematically related to the plane of the stimulated semicircular canal (see 'Central positional vertigo', below), which makes distinction from BPPV syndromes straightforward in most cases. The diagnosis is based on the temporal association of migraine symptoms. When a patient presents during a first episode of acute vestibular migraine, imaging may be required to exclude a central lesion, whereas a history of repeated episodes with complete remissions in between indicates a benign condition.

(For a more detailed description of vestibular migraine, see page 71 and Table 4.2.)

Central positional vertigo

Table 5.6 Central positional vertigo: key features

History	Prolonged (sometimes transient) vertigo, provoked by changes of head position Monophasic rather than relapsing/remitting course
Clinical findings	Positional testing should include supine head straight, head-lateral and head-hanging positions Variable combinations of nystagmus directions in the various positions possible; nystagmus usually persistent
Pathophysiology	Structural lesion of the vestibular nuclei or caudal cerebellum Abnormal central processing of otolith information
Investigations	Cranial MRI; further testing may be guided by MRI findings
Treatment	Directed at the underlying disorder

MRI = magnetic resonance imaging

Clinical features

Central positional vertigo is rare, accounting for fewer than 5% of patients presenting with positional vertigo. However, central positional vertigo usually indicates a structural lesion of the pontomedullary brainstem or caudal cerebellum which may become life-threatening in some patients. Therefore, a central disorder should be considered in all patients with positional vertigo.

Patients present with positional symptoms that may have existed for anything from a few hours to several years. The spectrum of complaints varies from positional vertigo, positional nausea or vomiting to positional oscillopsia (caused by positional nystagmus), all of which may occur in isolation or in combination. Sometimes central positional nystagmus is an incidental finding during clinical examination in a patient without positional symptoms but known neurological disease, such as cerebellar degeneration. Additional complaints such as double vision, slurred speech, incoordination or swallowing problems may point to posterior fossa disease early on in the course of investigation.

Clinical examination is most sensitive when nystagmus is observed not only in the classic Hallpike positions (Figure 5.1 on page 111; video clips 02.16 and 02.17) but also in the supine position with the head straight (nose up), head left and head right, and in the straight head-hanging position, i.e. with the head reclined 30 degrees from supine. Nystagmus direction and duration as well as subjective symptoms should be documented in all of these positions. Features suggestive of central positional nystagmus include:

- pure vertical (video clips 05.12 and 05.13) or pure torsional nystagmus with eyes straight ahead (video clip 05.14);
- oblique nystagmus (mixed vertical and horizontal);
- change of nystagmus plane with different head positions (e.g. from horizontal to torsional);
- persistent nystagmus (note that persistent horizontal apogeotropic nystagmus may be due to HC-cupulolithiasis-BPPV).

Associated neurological findings, especially brainstem and cerebellar signs, support a diagnosis of central positional vertigo (Table 5.7).

Pathophysiology

Lesions causing central positional vertigo are restricted to the structures around the fourth ventricle at the pontomedullary level: vestibular nuclei, cerebellar nodulus, and vestibulo-

Video 05.12 – Positional downbeat nystagmus
In this clip the patient is initially seen in the upright position and then immediately after reaching the left-ear-down Hallpike position. A downbeat nystagmus which takes several seconds to disappear is noted.

Video 05.13 – Positional downbeat nystagmus (video-oculography)
In this case the Hallpike manoeuvre was performed with a patient wearing an infrared oculography device. The video clip starts with reaching the head-down position. Soon after this a strong downbeat nystagmus develops which eventually disappears after a few seconds. The initial diagnostic impression was a midline cerebellar disorder but this was never confirmed on clinical or imaging examination and a provisional diagnosis of anterior canal BPPV was formulated.

Table 5.7 Brainstem and cerebellar signs associated with central positional vertigo

Abducens nerve palsy
Trigeminal hypaesthesia/pain
Facial paralysis
Dysphagia
Hoarseness
Gaze-evoked nystagmus
Defective-pursuit eye movements
Impaired VOR suppression
Gait ataxia
Dysarthria

Video 05.14 – Atypical (central) positional nystagmus
Same patient from video clip 03.05 – Pure torsional nystagmus, now shown during the Hallpike position with the left ear down. As the voice of the examining doctor indicates, the nystagmus is now beating in the opposite direction to the one observed in the upright position. In this case the patient is with the left ear down and the nystagmus is beating to the right, quite the opposite to what would be expected in BPPV. This patient has pontomedullary lesions of demyelinating origin.

cerebellar pathways. The aetiology of such lesions includes primary brain tumours and metastases, infarctions, bleedings, demyelination and local infections. Spinocerebellar ataxia type 6 often produces central positional vertigo and nystagmus as an early symptom. A more benign variant of central positional vertigo unrelated to structural pathology is caused by acute vestibular migraine. Positional downbeat nystagmus without concurrent vertigo often results from bilateral cerebellar disease such as cerebellar degeneration (see video clips 05.12 and 05.13). The exact mechanism of central positional vertigo and nystagmus is unknown. Persistent positional nystagmus most likely reflects abnormal central processing of otolith-derived head-position signals, whereas transient positional nystagmus may result from an exaggerated semicircular canal response. Both mechanisms may involve vestibular release from cerebellar inhibition.

Investigations
When central positional nystagmus is suspected an MRI should be performed. Further investigations such as cerebrospinal fluid (CSF) examination, vascular studies, search for a primary tumour or genetic testing depend on MRI findings and clinical presentation of the patient.

Differential diagnosis
A central lesion should generally be suspected when nystagmus features are atypical for BPPV or when brainstem or cerebellar signs are found. Isolated characteristics of BPPV like latency, duration and time course of nystagmus can also occur in central positional vertigo. However, it is unlikely that a central lesion mimics the entire nystagmus pattern of BPPV. The most reliable criterion to distinguish BPPV from central positional vertigo is the direction of nystagmus: when the affected canal is optimally stimulated in BPPV by specific head positioning in the canal plane, the nystagmus always beats in the plane which is expected from activation of that particular canal. Thus, in the Hallpike position, PC-BPPV always provokes a torsional nystagmus (with a minor vertical component) which is expected from the connections between the posterior semicircular canal and specific eye muscles. Likewise, horizontal canal benign paroxysmal positional vertigo evokes horizontal nystagmus of maximal intensity after specific positioning for the horizontal canal.

In contrast, central positional nystagmus is often not attributable to the stimulated canal plane. Purely vertical or torsional nystagmus, verified by examination under Frenzel's glasses, should raise the suspicion of a central origin, as it cannot be explained by stimulation of a single semicircular canal. Central positional nystagmus often persists as long as the precipitating head position is maintained and usually does not fatigue with repetitive positioning. Another feature that distinguishes central positional vertigo from BPPV is its monophasic course which makes the diagnosis highly unlikely in a patient with a long-standing history of recurrences and remissions. Vestibular migraine is the only recurrent vestibular disorder that may present with central positional vertigo and nystagmus.

In a patient with central positional vertigo and normal imaging, vestibular migraine or drug effects (e.g. amiodarone) should be considered. When central positional nystagmus without vertigo occurs as an isolated finding, imaging may be negative and a specific diagnosis cannot be made. One should remember that healthy individuals can show some positional nystagmus in total darkness.

Treatment

Therapeutic interventions are directed at the underlying disorder. In many patients the central positional nystagmus does not require specific treatment. For symptom control, vestibular suppressants and antiemetics can be used, but may fail in individual cases. In the acute stage, e.g. after stroke or demyelination, some patients need to stay in bed and keep their head still for several days. Parenteral nutrition may be transiently required. Positional exercises of any type are not helpful, but only aggravate the patient's symptoms.

Prognosis is variable depending on the pathological process. Patients with a persistent structural lesion may suffer from enduring positional vertigo and nausea since it is the central vestibular system itself that is damaged, making central compensation less likely. This is one of the rare causes of vertigo which requires long-term medication, starting with the least sedative substances.

Other causes of positional vertigo

Positional alcohol nystagmus and vertigo

This is not a real diagnostic challenge because most doctors have had some personal acquaintance of the intimate interaction between alcohol and the labyrinth. The nystagmus appears within 30 minutes after ingestion of alcohol whenever the patient turns his/her head to either side in the supine position. Positional nystagmus is horizontal with respect to the head and beats persistently towards the lower ear. It changes direction when the patient turns the head to the other side, beating again to the lower ear. This initial response decreases a few hours after alcohol consumption and is followed by a silent period lasting about two hours. Then positional nystagmus reappears with reversed direction, thus beating to the upper ear in each head-lateral position. Positional alcohol vertigo is explained by the fact that alcohol with its low specific gravity invades and leaves the endolymph and the cupula at a different pace, thus making the cupula first lighter and then heavier than the endolymph.

Perilymph fistula

A patient with a perilymph fistula may experience vertigo after changes of head position. There are conflicting data on the frequency of this manifestation. Detailed studies on the clinical features of positional vertigo and nystagmus are also lacking in these patients. Vertigo and nystagmus provoked by Valsalva manoeuvre during coughing, sneezing and lifting heavy objects is the more typical clinical presentation of a perilymph fistula (see page 88).

Vestibular paroxysmia or vascular compression of the eighth nerve

When neurosurgeons in the mid-eighties described the syndrome of vascular compression of the eighth nerve by a pulsating vessel they coined the term 'disabling positional vertigo'. At that time the variants of benign paroxysmal positional vertigo were not well delineated, and today it is rather doubtful if vascular compression accounts for a meaningful proportion of patients presenting with positional vertigo. Most attacks of vestibular paroxysmia occur spontaneously. Observation of a vessel crossing the vestibular nerve on MRI is certainly not sufficient to make the diagnosis, since asymptomatic contacts have been found in 20–30% of healthy individuals. A favourable response of vertigo attacks to carbamazepine is usually regarded as supportive evidence for the diagnosis.

For a more detailed discussion of suspected vestibular paroxysmia, see page 86.

Macroglobulinaemia, ingestion of glycerol and amiodarone intoxication

There have been single case reports of positional vertigo and nystagmus related to macroglobulinaemia, glycerol ingestion and amiodarone intoxication.

Head-extension vertigo: is it all cervicogenic?

Vertigo and imbalance that occurs while the head is extended is a clinical presentation only and does not imply a specific diagnosis. All too often, abnormalities of the cervical spine and muscles are suspected, leaving the real cause, often BPPV, untreated. One should remember that natural neck movements always involve concomitant head movement, thus stimulating vestibular receptors. The potential mechanisms of head-extension vertigo include physiological instability with head extension, PC-BPPV, any other positional vertigo, uncompensated vestibular disorders and, exceptionally, vertebral artery occlusion, carotid sinus hypersensitivity or the poorly substantiated concept of altered input from cervical mechanoreceptors.

Physiological instability with head extension

Every healthy person becomes somewhat unstable with the neck extended. For immediate evidence try this: stand on one leg with eyes closed. You may sway a little but you should manage. Now, try the same with your neck bent 45 degrees backwards. You will probably fall within a few seconds. This physiological instability can be explained by the fact that the vestibular organ is tilted 45 degrees out of its usual plane which requires a more complex analysis of incoming signals to adjust coordinates. In an unstable patient (e.g. with polyneuropathy), head extension may add that extra bit of imbalance that makes him fall.

PC-BPPV

This is the most common cause of vertigo after head extension and should be readily identified by positional testing. Positional testing can be performed without any neck extension, proving the labyrinthine rather than cervical origin of symptoms.

Any other positional vertigo

Horizontal canal BPPV and central positional vertigo can likewise cause vertigo upon neck extension. When Hallpike positional testing is negative, other positions should be tried, including lying in the nose-up, head-hanging and head-lateral left and right positions.

Vertebral artery compression

This is a rare cause of head-extension vertigo and usually requires not only head extension but also head rotation to trigger symptoms. Remember that a pulsating vessel erodes bone so that critical narrowing of the foramina transversaria is unlikely as long as the head is kept within the physiological range of movement. With extreme head positions, however, a vertebral artery can be compressed by osteophytes and muscles, which leads to vertigo when the opposite vertebral artery is hypoplastic. Vertigo and horizontal nystagmus can be provoked by head rotation, which needs to be maintained for at least 10 seconds. Dynamic angiography is needed to document the mechanism and site of occlusion (which is usually found at the C2 level). When avoidance of the offending head position is not possible or ineffective, surgery is indicated.

Carotid sinus hypersensitivity

Another extremely rare cause of head-movement-related dizziness is carotid sinus hypersensitivity. However, in order to document that this condition is truly responsible for the patient's dizziness, an ECG should be obtained during the usual provoking movement. A patient may well have sinus hypersensitivity under carotid sinus massage in the laboratory but his or her symptoms may result from BPPV.

Altered input from cervical mechanoreceptors

This is another potential mechanism for head-extension vertigo which is difficult to prove clinically if it exists at all. There is no doubt that muscle spindles in the upper neck provide somatosensory input to the vestibular nuclei, but the proven effects of local dysfunction on balance are far from impressive. Anaesthesia of the C2 nerve root in humans leads to transient gait problems but leaves balance during upright stance unaffected. Dizziness or vertigo after whiplash injury does not necessarily implicate cervicogenic vertigo but can be explained by various mechanisms, including dislodgement of otoconia from the otolith organs or other labyrinthine damage, BPPV, associated brainstem concussion or vertebral artery dissection.

To date, the concept of cervical vertigo has not been delineated as a clinical syndrome and specific tests to confirm the diagnosis are still lacking. Therefore, an effort should be made to find an alternative diagnosis which explains the patient's symptoms and which may be amenable to specific treatment. Associated neck pain may require physiotherapy nonetheless, and giving the patient the confidence to move the neck may ultimately promote compensation of an underlying vestibular disorder.

What to do if you don't have a clue

Occasionally, patients with positional vertigo may present in an atypical fashion. In the following we give some advice on how to manage difficult situations.

Testing impossible

Patients who are not willing to undergo positional testing can have two good reasons. Either they have been very sick with their attacks in the past or they have developed phobic avoidance of positional changes in response to the frightening experience of BPPV. The first should have an antiemetic before testing, while the latter should be either persuaded or sedated. Sometimes, both medication and a short admission to hospital are needed.

Negative Hallpike

A complaint of positional vertigo with negative positional tests can occur in different settings:

- The patient has experienced spontaneous remission days or weeks before he has managed to see you. Your waiting list is too long!

- You cannot provoke vertigo and nystagmus with the Hallpike manoeuvre, although the patient has been symptomatic until presentation. This may be due to horizontal canal BPPV which sometimes cannot be elicited by Hallpike testing. Try specific testing for the horizontal canals (see page 121). Another explanation is movement of the particles next to the canal wall which prevents relevant endolymph shifts while the particles are moving. Repeated testing in the same session or on another day is then likely to provoke nystagmus and vertigo. When the affected side can be inferred from the history, it is worthwhile doing an Epley or Semont manoeuvre. Alternatively, the clot causing BPPV may be lodged somewhere in the canal. Therefore, it is useful to repeat the manoeuvre with gentle head percussion or to see the patient again on another day. Remember also that being dizzy after getting up may implicate orthostatic hypotension rather than positional vertigo (see page 23, Figure 2.1).
- The patient complains of vertigo during positional testing but you don't see any nystagmus. Again, several causes are possible. There can be minimal BPPV that is not recognised during positional testing, especially when the patient cooperates poorly by moving his eyes all over the place. Studies have shown that doing a therapeutic manoeuvre for the symptomatic side is often beneficial in this situation. Then there are patients whose BPPV has disappeared spontaneously or after treatment, who feel some degree of positional vertigo when assuming the former offending position ('It is just about to come, but it does not really'). This may be a conditioned response to previous attacks, an erroneous expectation rather than true vertigo. This reaction can be unlearned with repeated positionings. Finally, introspective and anxious individuals may react intensely to the *physiological* vestibular sensation resulting from positional testing. When there is no nystagmus but an excessive behavioural reaction (sometimes causing hospital security to check the scene) you should start to explore the psychological dimension of the problem.

Who do you image?

In patients with typical BPPV no imaging is required. When BPPV is atypical, but otherwise neurological and eye-movement findings are normal, therapeutic positional manoeuvres can be tried for a week or two before MRI is requested. The yield of imaging will be low in this situation. However, when you feel uncomfortable with an atypical positional nystagmus, you may order a scan.

When neurological symptoms or signs, particularly those from the posterior fossa, are associated with positional vertigo and nystagmus, imaging should be performed immediately.

<table>
<tr><td>Chapter

6</td><td><h1>Chronic dizziness and unsteadiness</h1></td></tr>
</table>

Perhaps the most dreaded of all patients with balance disorders is the one with long-standing, continuous dizziness. If you are an ENT doctor this patient may have already seen a neurologist. If you are a neurologist your patient has definitely seen an ENT specialist. If you are a neuro-otologist the patient is likely to have seen both an ENT specialist and a neurologist. The patient almost certainly has had many sophisticated tests, including brain scans, audiograms, neck X-rays and maybe vestibular function tests. So, what are you going to do? It may be useful to separate this question into two: (a) what do patients with chronic dizziness have? and (b) what can you do for them? Table 6.1 lists the main conditions presenting with chronic dizziness and Table 6.2 provides an overview of the approach to this difficult patient.

Table 6.1 Chronic dizziness: diagnoses with key features

Main conditions are grouped as those with and without physical signs on examination. The conditions listed in the table are in no particular order of frequency, but we start with bilateral vestibular failure and the syndrome of downbeat nystagmus because they are often clinically missed.	
Condition or syndrome	Key features
Conditions with physical signs	
Bilateral vestibular failure (Page 141)	Bobbing oscillopsia when walking or driving. Unsteadiness worse in the dark. Bilaterally abnormal doll's head manoeuvre and head-impulse test. Vestibular tests useful
Downbeat nystagmus syndrome (Page 155)	Slowly progressive unsteadiness. Vertical oscillopsia. Downbeat nystagmus. Occasionally, additional cerebellar findings (e.g. speech)
Neurological gait disorders (Page 153, Chapter 7)	See Table 6.2: peripheral neuropathies; spinal cord syndromes (cervical myelopathy); cerebellar diseases (with/without downbeat nystagmus); cerebral disorders (parkinsonian syndromes, small-vessel white-matter disease)
Orthostatic Hypotension (Page 94, Chapter 4) (Page 150, Chapter 7)	Common in the elderly under antihypertensive drugs. Dizziness or pre-syncopal feelings whilst standing relieved by sitting/lying. BP drop on standing from supine (> 20mmHg, systolic)

Table 6.1 (*cont.*)

Condition or syndrome	Key features
Conditions with no physical signs	
Chronic vestibular migraine (Page 140)	Low-grade dizziness, nausea and migrainous features following recurrent vestibular migraine
Poorly compensated vestibular disorder (Page 132; under 'Patients with a past history of vertigo')	Residual dizziness after acute (Chapter 3) or recurrent (Chapter 4) vestibular event. Additional syndromes requiring special treatments are common (see PPD, Visual vertigo, this chapter)
Persistent perceptual dizziness (PPD) (Synonyms: phobic postural vertigo, chronic subjective dizziness, psychogenic dizziness) (Page 135)	Vestibular, general medical or psychological trigger ('I was fine until "this or that" happened'). Other medically unexplained conditions common. Minor vestibular findings possible but out of proportion with symptoms

The origin of chronic dizziness

Part of the problem in trying to understand what's wrong with chronic dizzy patients is that they can describe their problem in many ways. They can feel dizzy or giddy in the head, including sometimes mild rotational feelings, a bit 'drunk', detached, slightly off-balance or unsteady, that they seem to veer to one or both sides whilst walking, that they feel more steady if they touch or hold on to furniture, that they feel as if they were walking on a mattress or on cotton wool. These symptoms are fairly constant but there may be minor fluctuations, 'bad and good days'. We feel that the description of the *current symptom* is important but perhaps not as useful as the description of the *history of the symptom*. There are essentially three types of history: the patient who started with one or more attacks of rotational vertigo, the patient with a progressive history of disequilibrium, and the patient with neither of these.

PATIENTS WITH A PAST HISTORY OF VERTIGO

These patients report that at some time in the preceding months or years they suffered one or many vertigo attacks. Detailed history-taking should let you reach a retrospective diagnosis of vestibular neuritis, benign paroxysmal positional vertigo (BPPV) or other conditions discussed elsewhere in this book. In this case the patient will acknowledge that he or she does not currently suffer from disabling rotational vertigo but rather from a constant sensation of vague dizziness or subjective unsteadiness. If patients still report episodic vertigo attacks (e.g. BPPV, Ménière's disease, vestibular migraine, benign recurrent vertigo) they can easily distinguish between the acute recurrence and the chronic dizziness. In this case, the chronic dizziness tends to increase after each vertiginous episode.

Few published data are available but it is known that these patients are extremely common in specialised clinics. A patient who started with vestibular neuritis will describe that, say, 10 months ago he had the 'flu' and then severe vertigo nausea and imbalance for a week. He saw a doctor at that point and was told that he had a 'viral infection of the inner ear', that the symptoms would progressively go away and that he would return to normal or near normal within two to three months. Indeed, the majority of patients do recover fully within a few months, but a small proportion does not. Unfortunately, because acute and recurrent vertigo are so prevalent in the general population this 'small proportion' of patients make up considerable numbers of patients.

Table 6.2 Approach to the patient with chronic dizziness

Approach	Try to establish specific goals
Try to identify syndromes	Poorly compensated vestibular lesion (page 91) Visual vertigo (page 134) Motorist disorientation syndrome (page 135) Psychological disorder (page 135) Chronic vestibular migraine vertigo (page 140) Late-stage Ménière's disease (page 140) Bilateral vestibular failure (page 141) Neurological disorders (page 143)
Attempt retrospective diagnosis	Did it all start as BPPV, vestibular neuritis, brainstem stroke, migraine, Ménière's disease? Are the original symptoms still present? Or are we only dealing with chronic dizzy symptoms?
Multifactorial approach	Is vestibular compensation impeded due to additional problems? – Fluctuating vestibular disorder: recurrent vertigo – Visual problems: squints, cataract operation – Proprioceptive deficit: peripheral neuropathy (diabetes/alcohol) – Neurological problems: e.g. ischaemic white-matter disease – Orthopaedic problems and lack of mobility – Loss of confidence, fear of fall, psychological disorders – Age: all of the above possible, but try to identify which
Treatment is multidisciplinary	Treat any episodic vertigo specifically: – BPPV: repositioning manoeuvres – Vestibular migraine: migraine prophylaxis – Ménière's disease: radical or transtyrnpanic treatment Rehabilitation (and simple counselling): all patients Treat underlying complicating factors: e.g. orthopaedic, depression, diabetes Do not prescribe vestibular suppressants or tranquillisers (if you can, stop or reduce them)
Make sure the 'chronic dizziness' is not gait unsteadiness (Table 6.4, page 144)	'Is your problem a head or a leg problem?' Observe: gait, postural reactions and Romberg, eye movements and general neurological examination: Cerebellum: abnormal eyes, gait/limb ataxia Parkinsonism: resting tremor, increased tone, akinesia Spasticity: increased reflexes, Babinski sign Peripheral neuropathy: absent reflexes, distal weakness and sensory loss Frontal disorder/hydrocephalus/leucoaraiosis: gait 'ignition' failure, gait apraxia, shuffling, falls, cognitive problems Bilateral vestibular failure: unsteady gait with eyes closed; bilaterally abnormal doll's head and head-impulse manoeuvres

What can be happening here? Why do some patients not recover fully after one or more episodes of vertigo? We suspect that long-term symptoms are the consequence of some difficulty in the process of vestibular compensation. The process of central vestibular compensation is complex and it is often difficult to ascertain in each individual patient what may have interfered with the fine-tuning required to achieve full compensation. Possible causes are sometimes apparent, for instance if there are associated visual, peripheral nerve (proprioceptive) or central neurological problems, reduced mobility, or advanced age – which has all of the above. Often, however, the cause is not apparent and, in patients with anxiety, depression or other medically unexplained symptoms, one is tempted to attribute the chronic dizzy symptoms to a psychological problem; this will be discussed further under persistent perceptual dizziness (PPD), below. At the moment there is no definitive conclusion as to the exact mechanisms leading to chronic dizziness in patients with previous vestibular vertigo, but there is agreement that the problem is multifactorial and the solution multidisciplinary.

Some specific syndromes of patients with chronic dizziness have been described and, although the interpretation of these syndromes is still somewhat controversial, the reader will benefit from being familiar with the different modes of presentation in the clinic. Furthermore, regardless of the specific path into these syndromes, successful symptomatic treatments are available for them.

Visual vertigo

These are patients with chronic dizziness who report that their symptoms worsen in certain 'visually busy' surroundings. The syndrome is given different names, such as visual vertigo, visuo-vestibular mismatch, space and motion discomfort and, perhaps more accurately, visually induced dizziness. Frequently reported trigger situations are: walking through shelves in supermarket aisles (sometimes called the supermarket syndrome), viewing movement of large visual objects such as clouds, wind-swept trees, water flowing (river), disco lights, moving crowds, traffic, curtains being drawn, or films with car-chase scenes. Repetitive visual patterns like the stacks of cans in supermarket shelves, ironing striped shirts, or walking past a repetitive patterned fence also seem to be relevant. Some patients also mention that moving the eyes, reading and flickering or fluorescent lights can make them feel dizzy.

We know that, in many of the situations described, the visual environment contains too much information (e.g. the optokinetic stimulus provided by the supermarket shelves) or that the self-motion information conveyed by the visual and the vestibulo-proprioceptive systems are not in agreement. For example, movement of large visual scenes is normally interpreted as self-motion but in this case is not corroborated by (i.e. is in conflict with) the vestibular system (see 'Sensory conflict', page 15). We also know that all patients with vestibular lesions are prone to be influenced by visual stimuli, as part of the sensory substitution process that takes place during vestibular compensation. Furthermore, research has shown that patients with the visual vertigo syndrome are 'visually dependent'; that is, in them, vision is the predominant stimulus driving balance and spatial orientation. For these reasons, it should come as no surprise that intense visual motion stimuli and visuo-vestibular conflict can produce disorientation, imbalance and dizziness. Although the reasons why only some vestibular patients develop visual dependence and visual vertigo are not known, fortunately their symptoms can be improved by progressive exposure to visual motion stimuli and visuo-vestibular conflict during the rehabilitation programme (see Chapter 8).

Motorist disorientation syndrome

Driving, particularly on motorways (highways), can be uncomfortable for patients with chronic dizziness. Occasionally, patients report a sensation that the car is tilting or veering to one side. This sensation can be compelling, because often these patients see their mechanic or change their car before seeing their doctor. This 'motorist disorientation syndrome' also seems to be, at least partly, visually determined because patients describe problems in visually deprived areas (top of a hill or bridge), and in visually challenging conditions (e.g. simultaneously overtaking and being overtaken by a car). Indeed the coexistence of visual vertigo and motorist disorientation syndrome in the same patient is not rare.

Going round a bend, as when negotiating a roundabout, can also disorient patients but here there may be a predominantly vestibularly mediated mechanism. It must be kept in mind that driving through a curve is different from just turning round while walking. The radius of curvature is large while driving, so the conditions are equivalent to being centrifuged, and that is why you are pushed sideways against the door. In this case the unusual stimulation (sideways linear acceleration) acting on a damaged otolith system may be responsible for the symptoms. The additional, non-congruent, visual stimulation and the non-physiological posture, on vibrating cushions which numb somatosensory inputs, make driving a kind of sensory deprivation experiment in which vestibular asymmetries may re-emerge. Psychological components, usually in the form of panic and avoidance behaviour, can be contributory as well. In fact, in patients with no vestibular history or findings, a psychological disorder may be the only mechanism responsible. In these patients, however, there are usually more panic symptoms and less 'veering and tilting' of the car.

In patients with motorist disorientation syndrome comprising tilting-car illusions, previous history/findings of vestibular disease and no panic component, treatment will be based on vestibular rehabilitation including additional visuo-vestibular conflict and optic flow stimulation (see Chapter 8). In patients with predominant panic symptoms but no car-tilting illusions nor vestibular disease, treatment is psychiatric, often combining medication (e.g. SSRI, anxiolytics) with cognitive behavioural therapy.

Persistent postural perceptual dizziness (PPPD)

(Related terms: psychogenic/somatoform dizziness, phobic postural vertigo, chronic subjective dizziness)

In ancient medicine, vertigo and psychiatric symptoms were often regarded as the two faces of a single disorder originating from the brain. In contrast, modern medicine with its predominance of the natural sciences tends to neglect the psychological and behavioural dimension of vertigo and dizziness. However, emotions interact with orientation and balance in various ways, and differently in different people. For example, healthy people may feel quite uncomfortable, anxious and dizzy when they are exposed to heights. There are other individuals who feel and behave quite differently, including free climbers, parachutists or bungee-jumpers who are ready to risk their lives for the exciting experience of heights! Similarly, the emotional reaction of vestibular patients to their symptoms varies considerably, ranging from calm adaptation to the new situation to being 'frightened to death' by a vertigo attack. Interaction of mind and body may take the opposite direction as well: patients with purely psychiatric disorders often experience and express their distress with somatic symptoms such as chest pain, dyspnoea, diarrhoea, headache and, quite frequently, dizziness or vertigo.

Table 6.3 Key features of the syndrome of persistent perceptual dizziness (PPD)

History	Constant fluctuating dizziness and unsteadiness for more than three months; provocation by self-motion or exposure to moving visual stimuli Initially precipitated by acute or recurrent vestibular disorder, anxiety disorder or other medical condition
Clinical findings	Either normal examination or somatic findings which cannot fully explain the symptoms; often minor to moderate psychiatric abnormalities
Pathophysiology	Maladaptation to vestibular disorder or other stressful condition due to increased body vigilance, health anxiety and dysfunctional motor strategies
Investigations	Vestibular testing for assessment of somatic component or alternative diagnosis; psychiatric consultation
Treatment	Cognitive behavioural therapy; vestibular rehabilitation including exposure to visual motion and outdoor training Low dose SSRI in selected patients (?)

Clinical features

Persistent perceptual dizziness (PPD) is a new term that has been coined to integrate previous concepts such as *phobic postural vertigo, chronic subjective dizziness* or, more generally, psychogenic dizziness. It is the second most frequent diagnosis (after benign paroxysmal positional vertigo) in specialised dizziness clinics. The term PPD stresses the chronic nature of symptoms, while patients with panic disorder may have similar vestibular-like symptoms appearing in a paroxysmal fashion (see Chapter 4, page 99). The core of PPD is persistent non-vertiginous dizziness or unsteadiness on most days for more than three months. Anxiety, phobia or depression are commonly associated but may be lacking in individual patients.

The intensity of symptoms may fluctuate spontaneously or in response to provocative situations. Dizziness can be more severe when walking or standing and less intense when sitting or lying. Exacerbations may be prompted by active or passive self-motion, after a busy day, large-field visual stimulation, e.g. by cinema screens, moving crowds/traffic or supermarket aisles. Focused exposure to smaller visual targets, such as reading or computer work, may similarly induce symptoms. Many patients also react to classical agoraphobic stimuli such as leaving the house, crossing a large square and looking down from heights or to situations where they feel trapped, such as elevators, aeroplanes and queues at supermarket checkouts. Exacerbations may be superimposed by panic attacks (see Chapter 4, page 99) and can be accompanied by catastrophic thinking, e.g. an unfounded fear of falling. Instinctively, most patients avoid these provocative situations.

Thorough history-taking identifies an initial trigger in most PPD patients including a preceding vestibular disorder (e.g. vestibular neuritis, BPPV, Ménière's disease, vestibular migraine), mild traumatic brain injury or whiplash, panic attacks, generalised anxiety, orthostatic hypotension, cardiac dysrhythmia, syncope or medication side-effects.

Only a few other dizziness disorders, such as devastating brainstem or cerebellar lesions, can be as incapacitating in the long-term as PPD. Patients often feel unable to work, to leave the house unattended, to meet friends or to take exercise. Many depend totally on partners or other family members, some even stay in bed for most of the day.

Pathophysiology

The mechanism leading to persistent perceptual dizziness can be regarded as a maladaptive strategy to cope with a stressful event such as an acute vestibular disorder or a first panic attack with dizziness. These strategies are often useful at an early stage but become dysfunctional later on. For example, a cautious, small-stepped gait is completely appropriate for the acute phase of a vestibular illness, but detrimental when maintained longer than necessary. Conscious monitoring of balance or visual motion cues can be stabilising in the acute stage but may turn into a source of persistent irritation in the long run. Similarly, heightened awareness for body signals may be protective when health is acutely endangered but may also lead to misinterpretation of physiologic activity as imminent danger. Pre-existing anxiety and an introverted temperament may facilitate such maladaptive behaviours. Avoidance of provocative situations leads to even more anxiety and physical decline. All in all, PPD is not a purely psychiatric syndrome but rather results from a detrimental interaction of vestibular symptoms, psychological factors and dysfunctional behaviour (Figure 6.1).

Many patients with PPD report the syndrome described above as visual vertigo or visually induced dizziness. The underlying mechanism of visual vertigo is *visual dependency,* a strategy that relies predominantly on visual information for spatial orientation and balance with a relative neglect of vestibular and proprioceptive signals. Visual dependency may represent a personal trait, or it can be acquired in the course of a vestibular disorder where ignoring erroneous vestibular signals and putting more weight on visual cues can be, initially, an adequate strategy. The consequence of visual dependency, however, is detrimental because in the absence of a reliable reference, any movement of the visual environment may lead to self-instability and imbalance. In fact, patients with visually induced dizziness sway more than normal controls when they are confronted with moving visual scenes. Whether the visual vertigo is part of a poorly accomplished central vestibular compensation process, a pre-morbid high visual dependence or as part of a psychological trait present in PPD patients is not known. To some extent this question is mostly of academic interest because treatment with visual motion stimuli (see Chapter 8) seems effective for the visual vertigo component per se, regardless of the initial mechanism involved.

Clinical examination and investigations

Although clinical examination is mostly normal, there are many reasons why patients with suspected PPD should be carefully examined. Examination may reveal an underlying bilateral vestibular failure, downbeat nystagmus, residual levels of BPPV, peripheral neuropathy or other medical problems such as cardiac arrhythmia or postural hypotension. These conditions, which require treatment in their own right, may have triggered the development of PPD, but usually cannot fully explain the intensity of symptoms and the resulting handicap. Clinicians may refer to this as a degree of 'functional overlay'.

Another good reason to examine these patients and to perform laboratory tests is to gain their trust. They have come to see you as a dizziness doctor, not a psychiatrist. Unless they feel that you have the broad range of clinical skills required to make a diagnosis, manual and verbal, patients may not be open enough to discuss contributory emotional aspects. Formal psychiatric consultation can be useful for proper diagnosis of the psychiatric aspects

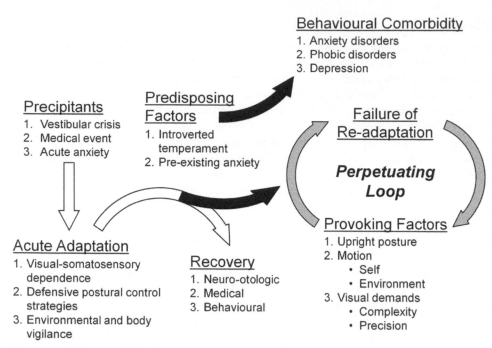

Behavioural Comorbidity
1. Anxiety disorders
2. Phobic disorders
3. Depression

Precipitants
1. Vestibular crisis
2. Medical event
3. Acute anxiety

Predisposing Factors
1. Introverted temperament
2. Pre-existing anxiety

Failure of Re-adaptation

Perpetuating Loop

Provoking Factors
1. Upright posture
2. Motion
 • Self
 • Environment
3. Visual demands
 • Complexity
 • Precision

Acute Adaptation
1. Visual-somatosensory dependence
2. Defensive postural control strategies
3. Environmental and body vigilance

Recovery
1. Neuro-otologic
2. Medical
3. Behavioural

Figure 6.1 Pathophysiology of persistent perceptual dizziness. Left: a precipitating event triggers an acute adaptation to maintain balance function. Normally, full recovery of neuro-otologic, medical and behavioural function is expected. On the background of predisposing factors, postural control systems may be pulled into a perpetual state of failed re-adaptation manifested by hypersensitivity to motion stimuli. Predisposing factors also increase the risk of developing psychiatric comorbidity. (Adapted from Staab 2012.)

and for specific treatment recommendations. Quite often, however, patients do not meet all diagnostic criteria of established psychiatric syndromes and their condition can be better understood by a dizziness doctor who knows about the behavioural consequences of vestibular disease. Finally a word of caution: do not order too many tests, as this may convey the message to your patient that he/she may still have a rare undiagnosed condition. Moreover, you will have to deal with false positive results or minor abnormalities which do not sufficiently explain the patient's condition. Do not deceive yourself and your patient by thinking that two to three tiny white spots in an MRI or a 10% caloric canal paresis explain major symptoms and psycho-social disability.

Treatment

How to inform patients about their condition? The patient's reaction depends, in our experience, largely on the doctor's ability to communicate and to establish a trustful relationship. Telling the patient 'it's all in your mind' is a very bad start. In any case, a potential negative reaction by the patient should not influence our diagnostic decision but rather prompt us to customise the wording when discussing the diagnosis with the patient. It is more important to convey the key messages to the patient than to use 'psycho' words. A good starting point can be the reassurance that health anxiety, cautious movements and avoidance of symptom-provoking situations are *normal* initial reactions to vestibular disease and other stressful events. The vicious cycle of high anxiety levels producing somatic symptoms which then lead to even more worry can be explained in simple terms. The patient usually agrees when the doctor supposes that the dizziness has gradually gained control over his/her life, telling him/her what to do and what to avoid. Most patients approve the therapeutic goal to regain their autonomy (unless some secondary gain hinders them). From there it is only a small step to the concepts of vestibular rehabilitation and cognitive behavioural therapy. These treatment approaches often need to be combined, particularly when patients have been off work for several weeks or months. Resuming sports and learning a relaxation technique such as progressive muscle relaxation should be encouraged because of their sympatholytic and anxiolytic effects. In addition, sports promote a sense of self-efficacy and body-confidence. Some patients, e.g. an elderly person with fear of falling, may not be able or may not wish to undergo psychotherapy. Vestibular rehabilitation can be even more effective in this situation as it ideally integrates physical training and psycho-behavioural interventions such as graded exposure to challenging tasks, reassurance and cognitive reframing (see Chapter 8, 'Rehabilitation').

When visually induced dizziness is a predominant complaint, vestibular rehabilitation should focus on visual desensitisation by exposing the patient to visual motion stimuli of increasing size and duration. This can be done by large-field optokinetic stimulation in a vestibular laboratory or by using a disco mirror ball. Alternatively, patients can be exposed incrementally to visual motion in their usual environments, including supermarkets, traffic and TV or computer screens.

Several open-label studies have shown that persistent perceptual dizziness may respond to serotonin-reuptake inhibitors. We are however cautious with respect to SSRIs because controlled studies are lacking and both their use and withdrawal may be associated with increased levels of anxiety. Treatment should follow a slow-and-low-regime, e.g. by starting with 5 mg of paroxetine with increases to 10 and 20 mg after two and four weeks. This approach makes full use of the placebo effect, which seems to be a major action of this class of antidepressants, while minimising side-effects such as nausea, sleep disturbance and sexual dysfunction. If the underlying disorder leading to PPD is vestibular migraine, 'old fashioned' tricyclic antidepressants such as amitriptyline taken at night may improve mood levels, promote better sleep and treat the migraine disorder prophylactically. As PPD patients are highly body-vigilant, one should minimise side-effects (mostly constipation, somnolence, dry mouth) by starting low and going slow.

Other psychiatric dizziness syndromes

Dizziness of psychiatric origin is found not only in anxiety disorders but also with depression and somatisation disorder. Dizziness due to depression is usually less dramatic in its presentation and is often described as a 'swimming sensation' or an inability to concentrate. It tends to be continuous rather than paroxysmal. Associated symptoms include depressed mood, lack of drive, fatigue, sleep problems and loss of appetite. Dizziness due to a depressive disorder usually disappears when the underlying illness is treated adequately with antidepressants or psychotherapy.

Somatisation disorder (formerly called hysteria or conversion disorder) is characterised by multiple and repeated somatic complaints and symptoms without an identifiable cause. These patients may present with a subjective complaint of dizziness only, or with non-organic ataxia, bizarre gait disorders or even an inability to stand in the absence of any abnormal neurological finding (Figure 6.2).

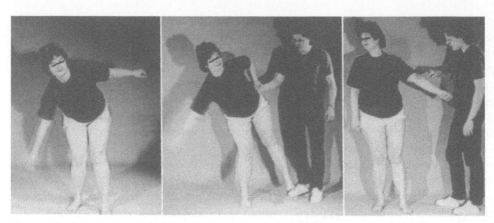

Figure 6.2 Somatisation disorder presenting with psychogenic pseudo-ataxia. Note the discrepancy of a swaying trunk in the presence of stable stance and the improvement by distraction while the patient is asked to recognise numbers written on her arm. (From: Lempert, Brandt, Dieterich, Huppert 1991, with permission of Springer Publishing.)

Chronic vestibular migraine

Like migraine itself, vestibular migraine presents with attacks rather than persistent dizziness (see page 71). A small subgroup of patients progresses from episodic vertigo at the beginning to chronic dizziness later on. At this stage, patients usually suffer from a constant seasick sensation of fluctuating intensity which is aggravated by head movement or visually challenging environments. Sometimes they also experience superimposed attacks of spontaneous or positional vertigo. Typical migraine headaches can be lacking but should be unearthed from the history by specific questioning. Again, enquiring about the early stages of the disorder is useful to make the diagnosis. Chronic vestibular migraine may be maintained or aggravated by psychological and behavioural factors, particularly anxiety, panic attacks, increased body-vigilance and avoidance of symptom-provoking situations. This syndrome has been designated as MARD: migraine and anxiety-related dizziness. The relative contribution of organic and behavioural factors is usually hard to disentangle in individual patients. Treatment often requires a combination of migraine prophylaxis (see Table 4.6, page 78), vestibular rehabilitation and cognitive behavioural therapy.

Late-stage Ménière's disease

Ménière's disease starts with episodic vestibular and cochlear symptoms, and there is complete resolution of symptoms in between attacks. As the disease progresses, patients develop permanent hearing loss and tinnitus and later sometimes also chronic dizziness and disequilibrium. After 10–15 years the attacks may eventually disappear while the chronic dizziness persists due to permanent damage to one or both labyrinths.

PATIENTS WITH PROGRESSIVE DISEQUILIBRIUM

Patients with progressive disequilibrium often present with a complaint of constant dizziness and it may take a few questions to understand that the problem is limited to standing and walking and disappears with sitting or lying down. Progressive disequilibrium is often caused by neurological disease and occasionally by bilateral loss of vestibular function, which deserves special attention as it often goes undiagnosed for many years. Therefore, it will be discussed first here.

Bilateral loss of vestibular function

This syndrome is caused by severe bilateral loss of vestibular function, and the symptoms arise as a result of loss of vestibulo-spinal and vestibulo-ocular reflexes. Bilateral vestibular failure (BVF) is not a rarity but, unfortunately, neither the average neurologist nor the average ENT surgeon is terribly familiar with this condition. If you think that your patient may have BVF and that your specialist colleague is not conversant with balance disorders you have two options: either develop the clinical skills yourself (with practice it is easy to diagnose this syndrome in an outpatient clinic), or refer the patient for vestibular tests or a neuro-otological opinion.

Aetiology

There are many causes of this syndrome. The most common are gentamicin otoxicity, post-meningitic, idiopathic and miscellaneous causes, these four groups being approximately equal in frequency. Some causes can be pretty obvious, such as post-meningitic BVF (patient usually deaf) or post-gentamicin intoxication (patient usually not deaf). Be aware that patients can undergo significant gentamicin vestibular toxicity, (a) with no hearing changes and (b) with normal serum levels of the drug, so a high level of suspicion is advisable. Other causes are less obvious, such as with the relatively common syndrome of idiopathic BVF. Some of these patients have also peripheral neuropathy and slowly progressive cerebellar signs suggesting a combined neurodegeneration. This combination is now called CANVAS: Cerebellar Ataxia, Neuropathy and Vestibular Areflexia Syndrome. There is preliminary evidence suggesting that some cases of idiopathic BVF are due to an ear-specific autoimmune disorder. Miscellaneous causes of BVF include generalised or cranial neuropathies, cerebellar degeneration, autoimmune disorders, bilateral 'burnt out' Ménière's disease and severe bilateral head trauma.

Clinical features

The syndrome of BVF, once fully established, is quite similar across patients with different aetiologies. Patients may seek help because of oscillopsia or unsteadiness, or often both. Since the oscillopsia is due to absence of the vestibulo-ocular reflex, patients will experience the visual difficulty during head or whole-body movements. Note that many patients may not spontaneously report movement of the visual world but just shimmering or blurring of images. Therefore, you have to ask whether the visual problem gets worse during riding in a car on a bumpy road or whilst walking fast and, reciprocally, if it gets better when the patient stops (video clip 02.01). Sometimes it is useful to say: 'Shake your head and look at me. Do I seem to jump or wobble around?' This often settles the matter.

The unsteadiness is made worse by walking in the dark, such as when going to the toilet in the middle of the night. Walking in the dark on a rough, irregular or compliant (yielding) surface is usually impossible and patients learn to avoid this or resort to a walking stick or holding on to someone's arm. Always enquire about unsteadiness in the dark in patients with oscillopsia, and about oscillopsia in patients whose unsteadiness worsens in the dark.

As part of the history-taking process you have to try to ascertain a possible aetiology behind the syndrome and how the patient reached the end-stage syndrome. A history of meningitis or ototoxic medication (particularly if there is renal dysfunction which interferes with drug excretion) will usually be volunteered, but don't take this for granted – enquire directly. These days the most common drug causing serious ototoxicity is gentamicin, but this usually causes little cochlear damage except in relatively rare genetic disorders (where patients get seriously deaf on minimal exposure to the drug).

Enquire about hearing loss and its time course. In systemic autoimmune and inflammatory disorders there is usually cochlear involvement, usually first on one side and then on the other. In patients with post-meningitic BVF and patients with ototoxicity the hearing loss develops in one single event. Some patients with bilateral Ménière's disease can develop BVF but they usually have a long history of tinnitus, recurrent vertigo plus fluctuating and progressive hearing loss.

The syndrome of idiopathic BVF has essentially three clinical presentations: repetitive episodes of brief paroxysmal oscillopsia, recurring vertigo attacks and progressive unsteadiness with oscillopsia in which patients gradually progress to the final chronic syndrome. These patients have no hearing symptoms.

Clinical examination

It is important to emphasise that except in cases of acute bilateral vestibular lesions such as meningitis or gentamicin intoxication, the syndrome of BVF is not as dramatic as you might expect. Most patients with idiopathic BVF walk in your consulting room uneventfully. In order to diagnose BVF you have to have a high index of suspicion.

The main abnormality of eye movements of the patient with BVF is due to the essentially absent vestibulo-ocular reflex (VOR) (see Chapters 1 and 2). Slow head turns from side to side whilst the patient fixates on your own nose or eyes (the doll's head-eye manoeuvre) will reveal 'broken up' or saccadic compensatory eye movements (instead of the purely slow-phase, smooth, compensatory VOR shown in video clip 02.12). The 'head-thrust' or 'head-impulse' test will reveal catch-up saccades after head movements both to the right and left (video clip 02.14). These manoeuvres are slightly more difficult to perform in the vertical (sagittal) plane but, if performed appropriately, vertical catch-up saccades will also be observed. Unless the BVF occurs in the context of a degenerative cerebellar disorder, where pursuit or saccadic abnormalities may be present, the remainder of the eye-movement examination is usually unremarkable.

As discussed in Chapter 2 (Figure 2.3), dynamic visual acuity is severely impaired in BVF so that a comparison of the patient's visual acuity during conventional static measurements and during head oscillation will reveal a discrepancy of two lines or more (e.g. from acuity 6/6 during static head to 6/36 during head oscillation). It is important that the doctor actively oscillates the patient's head, holding the head firmly from behind and 'shaking' it at 1–2 Hz. When patients move the head themselves they often stop or adjust the frequency/velocity so they can read properly, which may result in a false-negative result.

Loss of vestibulo-spinal function can lead to moderate to severe unsteadiness in the acute phase (e.g. after ototoxicity). However, it gradually improves as a result of vestibular compensation and increased reliance on visual and proprioceptive input. In a chronic, compensated state the conventional Romberg test is usually negative; that is, patients do not fall on eye closure. The tandem (heel-to-toe or sharpened) Romberg test and the one-foot

Romberg will be positive. Standing on rubber foam or a pillow, which degrades lower-limb proprioceptive input, with eyes closed, is usually impossible in patients with BVF. Gait with eyes open is often normal or slightly broad-based, but walking heel-to-toe or with eyes closed induces considerable unsteadiness.

Laboratory investigations
It is advisable to confirm the BVF with a formal vestibular test (either caloric or rotational), which will also quantify the magnitude of vestibular loss. In fact, the clinical manoeuvres described in the preceding section will be clearly positive only if the VOR loss is greater than 70–80% of its normal value. Imaging investigations are usually unhelpful. Blood tests, including syphilis serology and autoimmune screening, should be carried out but are usually normal.

Differential diagnosis
The differential diagnosis of BVF is broad and includes many disorders with gait unsteadiness and oscillopsia, in particular the downbeat nystagmus syndrome (see Tables 2.4, 6.2 and 7.5). If one can establish that the oscillopsia selectively appears during movement and the unsteadiness increases in the dark then the differential is quite narrow. Examination of eye movements, ruling out the presence of a central spontaneous or positional nystagmus (e.g. downbeat), is an important step. However, the single most significant step is documenting absent VOR during doll's head and head-thrust manoeuvres.

Treatment
The mainstay of treatment of the syndrome of BVF is rehabilitation. In fact, owing to the long delay usually incurred before a diagnosis of idiopathic BVF is made, most patients are partly self-rehabilitated for normal daily activities. However, even in these cases balance rehabilitation is helpful. As patients can feel devastated on learning that 'all inner-ear balance function has been lost', one should take the time to explain that in humans the inner ear only makes a small contribution to overall balance. Most patients continue to improve, from both the balance and oscillopsia symptoms, for several years after the insult. It is also important to warn patients about certain activities they should not carry out as they would expose themselves to serious risk, such as standing near the edges of cliffs or train platforms, snorkeling and scuba diving. The only good news for these patients is that, due to the absence of vestibular function, they have become virtually immune to motion sickness. Rarely, treatment for a possible underlying condition (e.g. autoimmune disorder) is needed. Steroids for the idiopathic cases cannot be recommended on current evidence.

Neurological disorders causing progressive disequilibrium
These disorders are dealt with in Chapter 7 (see page 153). It is appropriate to review the subject briefly here, because it is not always easy to separate patients with chronic dizziness following episodes of vertigo from those with gait unsteadiness, on the basis of the history alone.

Dizziness is usually described by the patients as a sensation in the head. They may say that they *feel* as if they were drunk but that, in contrast to true drunkenness, friends or

Table 6.4 Relevant questions and investigations in the patient with chronic disequilibrium

Associated symptoms	Suspected diagnosis	Investigations
Oscillopsia during head movement?	Bilateral vestibular loss	Head-thrust test, calorics
Persistent oscillopsia?	Downbeat nystagmus	MRI, cerebellar work-up*
Memory loss? Urinary urgency?	Hydrocephalus; cerebral small-vessel disease	CT or MRI
Numb, clumsy hands? Leg spasticity?	Cervical spondylotic myelopathy	Cervical MRI
Motor incoordination, dysarthria	Cerebellar ataxia	MRI, cerebellar work-up*
Distal numbness/weakness?	Polyneuropathy	EMG, biochemical tests
Slowness, akinesia, tremor?	Parkinsonism	Neurological consultation

MRI = magnetic resonance imaging; CT = computed tomography; EMG = electro-myogram
* Cerebellar work-up may include neurological consultation, alcohol history, MRI, general blood tests, thyroid function, vitamins B12 and E, inflammatory and paraneoplastic markers and possible genetic testing.

colleagues will not notice anything wrong with their balance. In contrast, the patient who describes disequilibrium due to gait unsteadiness will usually volunteer the information that loss of balance is noticed also by others. The patient may in fact have fallen or nearly fallen over as a result of the unsteadiness, again in sharp contrast to the patient with chronic dizziness secondary to a poorly compensated vestibular condition. In most cases, the disorders producing gait unsteadiness are progressive.

The diagnosis of the patient with disequilibrium is also heavily guided by the history, in particular the symptoms associated with the unsteadiness of gait. Table 6.4 provides a few questions that should help you in guiding the examination and type of laboratory investigations required. Note that MRI of the brain is not enough, and is definitely no substitute for a neurological examination in many of these conditions. The treatment of these disorders is part of general neurology and is mentioned only briefly in Chapter 7.

PATIENTS WITH NO HISTORY OF VERTIGO OR DISEQUILIBRIUM

Sometimes patients refer to a sense of vague and chronic dizziness with no history of 'true' vertigo nor disequilibrium. Direct general health questions may guide to disease of specific organs or systems (anaemia, thyroid, drug toxicity) but this line of enquiry is usually negative. A full clinical examination is warranted, including checking blood pressure supine and standing if the history suggests orthostatism.

This is a difficult patient group to diagnose and numerous investigations are often required, including blood tests to rule out general medical conditions such as anaemia, hypothyroidism or other endocrinological conditions, diabetes or hypoglycaemia, brain scans and vestibular function tests. With a history that is not disease-specific, an anxious personality and negative investigations, many patients are diagnosed as having psychogenic dizziness – rightly or wrongly. The acceptance of the concept 'persistent perceptual dizziness' (PPD see above) by the vestibular community has made the job of diagnosing psychogenic/psychosomatic dizziness somewhat easier. Observe, during history-taking, whether the patient appears to hyperventilate, and enquire about frank hyperventilation and anxiety episodes, as well as features that may indicate hyperventilation such as perioral paraesthesia. In our opinion, the active hyperventilation test is not so reliable because hyperventilation induces dizziness and unsteadiness in everybody, not only in patients with the hyperventilation syndrome. Only when the patient recognises his/her own typical symptoms during voluntary hyperventilation is the test useful. Blood gases and the opinion of a chest physician may be justified in some cases.

MANAGEMENT OF THE CHRONIC DIZZY PATIENT

Much of the management of the dizzy patient is presented in Chapter 8. We will summarise here the aspects specifically related to chronic dizziness.

Disease-specific treatment

If an active underlying vestibular disorder is identified, such as BPPV, migraine or Ménière's disease, this needs to be treated as outlined in Chapters 3–5. This is particularly important because with each vertigo attack the patient's chronic symptoms and anxiety tend to increase. By the same token, do not assume that if a patient is in a chronic phase he may not, for instance, have active BPPV. After months or even years of experience, patients with BPPV develop complex but 'effective' strategies to avoid the offending head positions and in extreme cases develop a phobia of lying down. In these cases if you find active BPPV you can treat it with the repositioning manoeuvres. If there is no BPPV you can begin to reassure your patient and thus engage him more diligently in an active rehabilitation programme. In summary, always try to establish whether your patient still has episodic attacks, and always examine your patient even if he or she denies having them.

Non-disease-specific pharmacological treatment

Vertigo or nausea can be improved with medication and these are very useful for the acute attack or the recurrent episode. Always enquire about medications your patient is taking. Most experts now believe that long-term use of vestibular suppressants and tranquillisers is counterproductive for the process of vestibular compensation. These drugs should be used only for the truly acute vertigo phase and stopped as soon as vertigo begins to recede, in a few hours or days. Explain briefly to your patients the process of vestibular compensation and that, for compensation to occur, the brain must feel *some* vertigo. This sensation functions as a warning signal driving the compensation processes. Explain that no vertigo at all means no warning signal, and hence no compensation.

Sometimes it is difficult to wean patients off medication they may have taken for a long time and one has to compromise and let the rehabilitation begin before complete medication withdrawal.

Patients with migraine or vestibular migraine overusing pain killers will benefit from switching on to prophylactic medication (see Chapter 4, page 78). It may be useful to implement this switch before starting the rehabilitation process, as migraine symptoms may initially increase during the eye, head and visual motion exercises required.

General support

Reassurance, information and counselling are extremely important (see Chapter 8). Explain in simple terms the process of vestibular compensation and that sometimes, with or without obvious reason, compensation is incomplete. Provide useful web-pages or leaflets, explain the need for rehabilitation, and try to motivate your patients to participate actively in their own recovery process (see 'Further reading', page 184).

Rehabilitation

In this chronic group, rehabilitation is the most important aspect of the treatment. The complexity of the rehabilitation offered to the patient will depend on two factors:

- how much, if any, rehabilitation and advice your patient has already had;
- how much access you have to (and how good is) your rehabilitation team.

For the patient who has been (ill-)advised to stay in bed and take tablets when he is dizzy, simple explanations, counselling to begin activity and a progressive reduction in medication may be enough. The other end of the spectrum is the patient who has already done a course of conventional vestibular rehabilitation but has developed visual vertigo and psychological complications. This patient may need specialised vestibular rehabilitation including optic flow techniques. Although there is considerable variation, according to medical practices in different regions and countries, most chronically dizzy patients are likely to be in between these two extremes.

The detailed assessment and treatment aspects of rehabilitation can be found in Chapter 8. The majority of the discussions offered there, in particular as to counselling and psychological presentations, are highly relevant to the chronic patient. Most patients will have psychological complications. Separating 'organic' from 'psychogenic' or 'primary' from 'secondary' is deeply engrained in our medical training, but nowhere is it more difficult to separate these than in patients with chronic dizziness. The effort to distinguish organic from psychogenic may not always be worthwhile and many patients are willing to undertake additional cognitive behavioural or other psychotherapies if they see this as part of a global 'body and soul' effort. Some patients may need antidepressant medication, particularly on initiating the rehabilitation process. Although there is no evidence one way or another, the consensus is that antidepressants do not interfere with vestibular compensation or rehabilitation.

What to do if you don't have a clue

- Do not miss underlying neurological disease – consider neurological referral.
- Do a positional test, even if the history does not sound like BPPV. You may find BPPV or positional downbeat nystagmus.
- Watch out for bilateral vestibular failure, enquiring about oscillopsia during head movements and by doing the head-thrust test and the VOR reading test (see page 36).
- Enquire about chronic migraine features (low-grade headaches, photophobia, nausea). Migraine and dizziness feed off each other and migraine prophylactic treatment may provide the first stepping stone in the path to recovery.
- Pay attention to psychological aspects such as stressful life events, anxiety or medically unexplained symptoms and depression which may cause or aggravate the problem.
- If there is a past history of vertigo, even when the current diagnosis is unclear, most patients will benefit from vestibular rehabilitation.

Dizziness, imbalance and falls in the elderly

Introduction

Dizziness in elderly patients is so common that it is often dismissed as a normal age-related phenomenon. Alternatively, neck problems or atherosclerotic vessels are blamed even before any detailed history has been taken and a clinical examination performed. However, just like in younger patients, your primary goal should be to find the underlying cause of the patient's symptoms which may lead the way to specific treatment (Table 7.1). Nevertheless, many elderly patients do not have a single identifiable disease but rather a multitude of medical conditions which may cause dizziness and imbalance. Therefore, identification of

Table 7.1 Dizziness in the elderly: diagnoses with key features

Disorder	Key features
Effects of physiological ageing (page 148)	Chronic (and mostly mild) imbalance and dizziness due to age-related decline of vestibular, somatosensory, visual and motor function
Drug-induced dizziness (page 149)	Permanent, fluctuating or episodic dizziness caused by various mechanisms: sedation, vestibular suppression, ototoxicity, cerebellar toxicity, orthostatic hypotension, hypoglycaemia
Benign paroxysmal positional vertigo (page 149)	Brief attacks (< 30 s), provoked by turning in bed, lying down, sitting up from lying, head extension or bending over Symptomatic episodes for weeks to months, remissions for years Mainly torsional nystagmus beating towards the ground in lateral head-hanging position
Orthostatic hypotension (page 150)	Episodes of dizziness on standing up or staying upright Relieved by sitting/lying down Drop of systolic blood pressure of $\geq$ 20 mmHg after standing up
Vascular disorders (page 151)	Symptoms are related to localisation: • Labyrinthine TIA/infarction: vertigo with hearing loss • Brainstem TIA/infarction: vertigo with neurological symptoms • Widespread white-matter lesions: chronic imbalance and dizziness. Falls possible
Neurological disease (page 153)	May cause dizziness and imbalance when locomotor sensory or motor systems are affected, e.g. polyneuropathy, myelopathy, Parkinson's disease, cerebellar disease (including downbeat nystagmus syndrome), hydrocephalus

Table 7.1 (cont.)

Disorder	Key features
Fear of falling and cautious gait (page 158)	Small stepped gait in the absence of a relevant neurological or vestibular disorder
Cardiac arrhythmia (page 158)	Dizziness lasting seconds; may be accompanied by palpitations; can be caused by bradycardia < 40/min or tachycardia > 170/min.
Orthopaedic disorders (page 159)	Hip and knee problems before and after replacement surgery

TIA = transient ischaemic attack

contributing factors to the patient's dizziness should complement the search for a specific diagnosis. This may be illustrated by a clinical example.

> A 78-year-old lady enters the consultation room: 'I am always dizzy, doctor' (which is probably the most popular opening phrase in neuro-otology). On questioning, she specifies that the sensation of dizziness is related to imbalance whenever she is standing and/or walking, particularly in the dark, whereas during sitting or lying she is symptom-free. The onset of symptoms has been gradual over the past two years and she has never experienced any vertigo or nausea. When standing up after meals she often feels light-headed and has fainted twice. Type 2 diabetes was diagnosed 10 years ago and hypertension 6 years ago, and treated since then. She has undergone hip replacement surgery on the right nine months ago. Previous caloric testing and ultrasound of the neck arteries has been normal. She brings an MRI scan of the brain which is normal except for multiple small white-matter lesions in the cerebral hemispheres.
>
> Examination, including positional testing, shows no vestibular signs, but there is imbalance on Romberg testing which worsens after eye closure. Tandem walking is somewhat unstable and she staggers when she turns around. There are no cerebellar signs. Ankle jerks are absent on both sides. Proprioception (joint position sense and tuning fork), touch and pinprick sensation are severely impaired in her feet. Hip movement on the right is painful and restricted to 45 degrees of flexion and 10 degrees of extension. Orthostatic blood pressure, measured after the patient had a meal at the hospital cafeteria, shows a drop from 130/85 mmHg (supine) to 90/50 mmHg (standing) with concurrent light-headedness and faintness.
>
> In summary, this patient has two types of dizziness: one is related to poor balance and the other to postprandial orthostatic hypotension. The balance disorder is multifactorial with diabetic neuropathy as the main component and subcortical ischaemic lesions, decreased hip mobility and age as contributing factors. Postprandial hypotension is common in elderly hypertensive patients and is probably aggravated by autonomic diabetic neuropathy and anti-hypertensive agents in this patient.

In the following we will discuss disorders that often cause dizziness or vertigo in the elderly. Some of them, such as drug side-effects, benign positional vertigo and orthostatic hypotension, can be effectively treated, if they are thought of and searched for by specific clinical testing.

Effects of physiological ageing on balance

It is common knowledge that balance, like memory, is poor in the elderly. Balance is a process dependent on a number of peripheral sensory inputs (chiefly proprioceptive, visual and vestibular) which are integrated centrally and combined with other neural functions such as motor control and cognition. It is well documented that the elderly show loss of function in each of these sensory modalities and each of the central processes required. Furthermore, there are usually good correlations between variables measured, such as age-related loss of a peripheral proprioceptive sensitivity and increase in postural sway. In addition to a decrement in sensory receptor sensitivity, as well as peripheral and central neural function, the elderly also show non-neural changes that impinge on balance control – such as vascular and osteo-articular factors.

From the point of view of the clinician, 'criteria of normality' have to be adjusted when examining an elderly patient. Three daily encountered examples, notably relevant for balance function, are loss of ankle jerks, decreased vibration sense in the ankles and decreased-pursuit eye movements. The first two illustrate the loss of large-fibre input to stretch reflex mechanisms and proprioception, whereas the latter (pursuit) points to the loss of midline cerebellar function in the elderly. The implications are threefold:

1. As mentioned, normal clinical criteria have to be adjusted. For example, the isolated finding of abnormal pursuit does not indicate a central vestibular disorder as it would in a young patient.
2. The so-called 'normal age-related clinical findings' testify to the underlying mechanisms responsible for the physiological decrement in balance in the elderly – even in the absence of disease.
3. Any additional disease process affecting balance, such as a peripheral vestibular disorder, will have a larger impact in an elderly patient. Similarly, the process of recovery (e.g. 'vestibular compensation'), typically relying on sensory substitution and central compensation, will be compromised.

Drug-induced dizziness

Most elderly people in industrialised countries take drugs on a regular basis, often five or more at a time. Aggressive pharmaceutical marketing, unnecessary prescriptions, ignorance of possible drug interactions and disregard for altered drug metabolism in the elderly all add to iatrogenic morbidity in the form of drug-related adverse effects – with dizziness ranking among the most common. Several drug effects, such as sedation, slowing of reaction time and imbalance, may promote falls. Indeed, a statistical association between drugs and falls has been established for benzodiazepines, tricyclic antidepressants, serotonin-reuptake inhibitors and acetylcholinesterase inhibitors (for treatment of Alzheimer's disease). Drug-induced symptoms may fluctuate with rising and falling plasma levels or may persist either when high plasma levels are maintained or when permanent damage has been inflicted. Again, it is worthwhile trying to differentiate between various types of dizziness which reflect the diverse underlying drug-related mechanisms involved (Table 7.2). For a more detailed description of these mechanisms refer to Chapter 4, page 102.

Benign paroxysmal positional vertigo (BPPV)

This is a condition characterised by brief episodes of vertigo that are provoked by changes of head position (see Chapter 5). The diagnosis is confirmed when Hallpike positional testing provokes typical nystagmus (video clips 02.17 and 05.01). BPPV is caused by displaced otoconia which have entered a semicircular canal where they provoke endolymph

Table 7.2 Symptoms, signs and mechanisms of drug-induced dizziness

Symptoms/signs	Mechanism	Sample drug
Imbalance, drowsiness, poor concentration	Sedation	Diazepam, alprazolam phenobarbitone
Imbalance, drowsiness, poor concentration	Vestibular suppression	Dimenhydrinate, promethazine, diazepam
Imbalance (worse in the dark), oscillopsia during head movement, bilateral VOR loss	Ototoxicity	Gentamicin, streptomycin, cisplatin
Gait and limb ataxia, dysarthria, gaze-evoked nystagmus	Cerebellar toxicity	Carbamazepine, phenytoin, lithium
Orthostatic dizziness, blackouts, syncope	Orthostatic hypotension	Nitroglycerine, furosemide, propranolol, captopril, amitryptiline, L-dopa, tamsulosin

VOR = vestibulo-ocular reflex

shifts whenever the head postion is changed (for details, see page 109). Otoconia may dislodge from the otolith organ secondary to trauma, labyrinthine disease and age-related degeneration. Therefore, idiopathic BPPV becomes more prevalent with advancing age, whereas the (less common) symptomatic forms of BPPV do not. Population-based estimates on the frequency of BPPV across various age groups show an increasing prevalence in the elderly reaching 10% in people over 80. This figure provides sufficient justification for routine Hallpike testing in all dizzy patients aged above 60. We have seen quite a few older patients who denied any positional vertigo even on specific questioning and then had typical vertigo and nystagmus on positional testing.

Treatment of BPPV can be difficult in the elderly for several reasons. Patients with decreased neck mobility may have problems achieving sufficient head rotation and reclination as required for the Epley manoeuvre (see Figure 5.3 and video clip 05.04). In this case, one can use an examination couch where the head portion can be lowered by 30 degrees so that both trunk and head are reclined during treatment and further reclination of the head is not required. Alternatively, one can apply Semont's manoeuvre which does not involve any head reclination (see Figure 5.4 and video clip 05.02). On the other hand, frail or obese patients may not be able to cooperate during the rapid body swing involved in Semont's manoeuvre. Performing the manoeuvre is much easier when a second therapist supports the patient from behind; your outpatient nurse can do this if you offer minimal training. Finally, concurrent cognitive problems may interfere with understanding and performing self-treatment at home (see Figure 5.5). Therefore, correct execution of the self-paced manoeuvre should be checked during consultation.

Orthostatic hypotension

Orthostatic hypotension affects 5–30% of elderly individuals. Specific risk factors in old age include hypertension, congestive heart failure, dehydration and medications such as antihypertensives, diuretics, tricyclic antidepressants, tamasulosin (sutiprostate) and antiparkinsonian drugs.

By definition, orthostatic hypotension requires a drop of at least 20 mmHg systolic or at least 10 mmHg diastolic blood pressure after standing up. Unfortunately, measurement of orthostatic blood pressure is burdened with false-positive and false-negative results. Quite a few elderly patients with orthostatic hypotension have no orthostatic symptoms and do not require treatment (false positives). On the other hand, symptomatic orthostatic hypotension may go unnoticed (false negatives) when measurements are taken at random times and not when an individual patient is usually symptomatic, such as in the morning, after meals or after dialysis. Therefore, diagnosis should be based on the combination of a positive orthostatic history and a positive orthostatic blood pressure test performed at the appropriate time. Repeated measurement may be necessary in doubtful cases. For treatment of orthostatic hypotension, see page 96.

Vascular disorders

Atherosclerosis is common in elderly subjects, but exactly how vascular disease causes dizziness and vertigo in the elderly deserves consideration. 'Vascular vertigo' is neither a distinct disease nor even a syndrome but rather a category that includes various disorders which differ in localisation, pathophysiology and clinical presentation.

Labyrinthine transient ischaemic attack or infarction

This typically presents with acute spinning vertigo and profound hearing loss due to cochlear involvement. Isolated ischaemia of the vestibular labyrinth is theoretically possible but appears to be rare (see Figure 1.5). On examination, there are signs of acute unilateral loss of labyrinthine function: spontaneous horizontal–torsional nystagmus beating towards the intact side (e.g. left-sided deafness and a right-beating nystagmus), a pathological head-impulse test during head rotation towards the affected side, a pathological Romberg with swaying towards the affected side and unilateral deafness.

Infarction of the root entry zone of the eighth nerve

Ischaemia at this site is very rare and may mimic vestibular neuritis. Suggestive features include advanced age, vascular risk factors, sudden onset and variably associated neurological signs such as skew eye deviation, saccadic pursuit, Horner's syndrome, facial palsy or ipsilateral limb ataxia.

Brainstem/cerebellar transient ischaemic attack or infarction causing vertigo

Acute vascular vertigo commonly results from ischaemia in the territory of the anterior or posterior cerebellar artery, or from partial lesions restricted to the brainstem or pontomedullary junction. The critical structures are the vestibular nuclei and the vestibulocerebellum which inhibits the ipsilateral vestibular nuclei (see page 60).

Cortical transient ischaemic attack or infarction

This is an exceptionally rare cause of vascular vertigo and requires involvement of the core area of the multimodal vestibular cortex in the posterior insula and temporoparietal junction.

Small-vessel disease affecting the pons

Scattered vascular lesions in the pons have been identified as a quite common cause of chronic imbalance. In the pons, fibres from the motor cortex are relayed to the cerebellum via the pontine nuclei. Small-vessel disease in this area may lead to patchy vascular demyelination which is visible on T2-weighted magnetic resonance imaging (Figure 7.1).

Small-vessel disease affecting the cerebral white matter

Small-vessel disease causes imbalance when multiple periventricular lesions affect sensory and motor fibres connecting the cortical leg areas with the thalamus, basal ganglia, cerebellum and spinal cord (video clip 07.06). Severely affected patients have additional features such as pseudo-parkinsonian gait, incontinence and subcortical dementia. Typically, patients have long-standing hypertension and sometimes diabetes. The neurological examination may reveal focal signs such as hemiparesis, spasticity or extensor plantar responses. MRI shows enlarged perivascular spaces in the basal ganglia and cerebral white matter, lacunar infarctions and patchy or confluent T2-hyperintense white-matter lesions resulting from vascular demyelination (Figure 7.2).

As these changes reflect permanent ischaemic damage to the brain, treatment options are limited. Antiplatelet agents such as aspirin and clopidogrel have no proven effect on slowing the progression of cerebral small-vessel disease. Hypertension and diabetes should be controlled, although aggressive treatment may cause additional damage due to repeated hypoperfusion and hypoglycaemia. The authors believe that the combination of small-vessel disease and postural hypotension is a leading cause of dizziness in the elderly. Physiotherapy with gait and balance exercises may enhance the patient's residual function. Often, walking aids are needed.

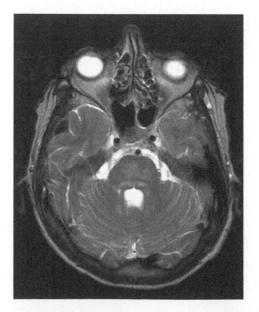

Figure 7.1 Vascular demyelination of the pons in a patient with chronic imbalance.

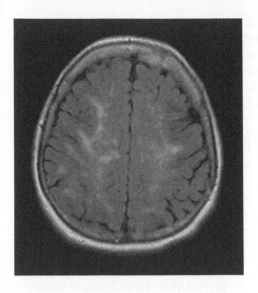

Figure 7.2 Subcortical small-vessel disease on T2-weighted MRI.

Multiple cerebral infarctions

Infarctions due to repeated cardiac embolism or severe atherosclerosis will cause chronic imbalance when critical sensory and motor structures are involved: dorsolateral thalamus, the paramedian leg areas of the motor cortex, basal ganglia, cerebellum and the fibre tracts connecting these structures. Additional neurological deficits which are commonly associated include paresis, sensory deficits, aphasia and dementia.

Neurological disease

Progressive unsteadiness with dizziness is often caused by non-vascular neurological disease in the elderly. It may result from motor or somatosensory dysfunction at any level of the nervous system from the peripheral nerves up to the brain. Common conditions include polyneuropathy, myelopathy, cerebellar disorders, Parkinson's disease and hydrocephalus.

Polyneuropathy

Usually, the first symptom of polyneuropathy is tingling or numbness in the feet. Some patients, however, present with a primary complaint of unsteadiness which worsens in the dark, and distal sensory loss may become evident only on clinical examination. The most sensitive sign of peripheral neuropathy is often diminished vibration sense in the toes and ankles but this finding is not uncommon in the elderly without clinically relevant poly-neuropathy. Hence, absent vibration sense at the top of the shank is a more convincing sign. A significant sway increase on eye closure during the Romberg test (video clip 07.01) may appear long before a decreased sensation to touch and pin-prick are noted. Most neuropathies start with sensory symptoms but distal weakness (toes, ankles) may develop later on. Of particular relevance to balance is the ankle extensor weakness encountered in many neuropathies as these muscles are responsible for toe clearance during forward swinging of the leg during locomotion. Weakness of these muscles leads to falls as the toes get caught during walking. Electromyography with low amplitudes of sensory or motor action potentials or decreased conduction velocity will confirm the diagnosis.

An aetiology can be found in about 70% of patients, with diabetes and alcohol abuse accounting for at least half of them. Always probe your patients for alcohol intake if you suspect the presence of polyneuropathy. Other causes include hereditary neuropathies, vitamin deficiency (e.g. B1, B6 or B12), inflammatory and autoimmune disorders (vasculitis, rheumatologic diseases, paraproteinaemia, Guillain–Barré syndrome, chronic inflammatory demyelinating polyneuropathy), renal failure, chronic liver disease, paraneoplastic disorders (particularly with small-cell carcinoma of the lung), toxins (e.g. organic solvents) and medications (e.g. vincristin, cisplatin, paclitaxel, phenytoin, amiodarone). An initial work-up should include fasting blood glucose, HbA1c, renal and liver function tests, blood count, ESR, antinuclear antibodies, immune electrophoresis and B12. For patients with subacute neuropathy developing within weeks, a search for occult malignancy including antineuronal antibodies is advisable. Once the cause of neuropathy is known, specific treatment (or elimination of toxins) may lead to remission of the neuropathy or at least retard its progression.

Myelopathy

While acute disorders of the spinal cord usually present with flaccid paraparesis and a sensory level, chronic myelopathy is often characterised by progressive spasticity, before weakness and sensory dysfunction become evident. Consequently, patients complain about gait problems with stiffness/heaviness in their legs and it takes a thorough neurological examination to detect extensor plantar responses, increased tendon reflexes, spasticity and (sometimes subtle) sensory dysfunction in the legs. In the absence of a sensory level the lesion may be difficult to localise and MRI of both the cervical and thoracic cord may be required. However, involvement of the hands (e.g. wasting of hand muscles or numb fingers) clearly points to the cervical cord.

Common causes include cervical spondylotic myelopathy, tumours such as meningioma or low-grade glioma, and primary progressive multiple sclerosis which often manifests itself with a purely spinal syndrome. In populations with dizziness and unsteadiness as presenting symptoms, cervical spondylotic myelopathy is by far the leading spinal cord disorder as it affects mostly elderly patients, sometimes as one element of a multifactorial balance disorder. The archetypical patient would be about 70 years old and complaining about gait problems and numb, clumsy hands. MRI visualises narrowing of the cervical spine, most often at the C5/C6 level. T2-hyperintensities within the cord at the level of compression indicate secondary ischaemic damage, which is usually permanent. As always, a combination of clinical and radiological findings is required for diagnosis – and even more so for surgery. Moderate and even severe radiological appearances without concomitant neurological findings are unlikely to explain your patient's imbalance.

Unfortunately, scientific evidence to guide management is weak. Retrospective studies have shown that conservatively treated patients are often stable for years, while some deteriorate at a fast pace. Surgery is commonly advised when spinal narrowing causes neurological problems, particularly when symptom progression is fast.

Video 07.01 – Sensory neuropathy: Romberg test
This patient with advanced sensory neuropathy becomes severely unstable after eye closure (positive Romberg test).

Cerebellar disorders

The symptoms of cerebellar disease can be attributed to the three subsections of the cerebellum: ataxia of the extremities and dysdiadochokinesis reflect dysfunction of the cerebellar hemispheres; gait and truncal ataxia result from involvement of midline structures (cerebellar vermis); while ocular motor signs such as saccadic pursuit, gaze-evoked nystagmus, impaired VOR suppression and downbeat nystagmus point to the caudal cerebellum (flocculus and paraflocculus) (video clips 02.22–02.24). Neurological disorders commonly affect various parts of the cerebellum so that a mixture of symptoms is found in most patients. When looking at the cerebellum from the perspective of progressive unsteadiness we are dealing with chronic disorders (for acute cerebellar lesions see page 60).

The differential diagnosis includes hereditary degeneration, sporadic degenerations such as the cerebellar type of multiple system atrophy, Chiari malformation, multiple sclerosis, tumours such as haemangioblastoma or meningioma, alcohol abuse, hypothyroidism and paraneoplastic cerebellar degeneration (which progresses rapidly over weeks).

Magnetic resonance imaging is required to detect cerebellar lesions or atrophy and to search for associated findings such as brainstem atrophy in multiple systems degenerations or periventricular demyelination in multiple sclerosis. Blood tests including cell count and morphology, liver function tests, thyroid function, vitamin levels (B12, folate, E), inflammatory and tumour markers can be helpful. Genetic testing for identification of one of the about 45 subtypes of autosomal dominant spinocerebellar ataxia (SCA 1, 2, 3, etc.) is useful if there is a suggestive family history or if the risk for relatives and offspring needs to be assessed. In patients with midline cerebellar symptoms, including gait and eye-movement signs such as spontaneous or positional downbeat nystagmus, the SCA 6 gene mutation is occasionally found.

Degenerative cerebellar disorders are not amenable to medical treatment with the exception of episodic ataxia type 2, which often responds to acetazolamide or aminopyridines. Physiotherapy, in particular intensive coordination training, has some effect on gait and extremity ataxia, particularly when there are no associated sensory deficits.

Downbeat nystagmus syndrome deserves special consideration for several reasons. It presents fairly selectively to balance clinics and it is a relatively common condition – many new patients are seen every year which the authors can testify have been missed in general neurology and ENT clinics (video clips 07.02, 07.03 and 7.04). Patients complain of slight unsteadiness and sometimes vertical oscillopsia or vague visual dysfunction. Detection of downbeat nystagmus in the primary position requires close

Video 07.02 – Downbeat nystagmus
The video clip shows a patient with slight downbeat nystagmus in primary gaze which is enhanced by convergence and on gaze deviation to the right and the left. More video clips of the same patient: 07.03 – Gait in a patient with downbeat nystagmus, and 07.04 – Finger – nose test in a patient with downbeat nystagmus.

Video 07.03 – Gait in a patient with downbeat nystagmus
The video clip shows the patient with a downbeat nystagmus/gait ataxia syndrome trying to walk on a narrow base. Note that he tends to step outside the mark indicated on the floor and that he is unsteady on turning. More video clips of the same patient: 07.02 – Downbeat nystagmus and 07.04 – Finger – nose test in a patient with downbeat nystagmus.

Video 07.04 – Finger – nose test in a patient with downbeat nystagmus
The video clip shows the finger – nose test in a patient with downbeat nystagmus and gait unsteadiness. Note that the finger – nose test is essentially normal. More video clips of the same patient: 07.02 – Downbeat nystagmus and 07.03 – Gait in a patient with downbeat nystagmus.

inspection and sometimes magnification by funduscopy (remember that you will see the eye beating up through the ophthalmoscope as you are looking at the back of the eye). The downbeat nystagmus typically increases during convergence and on lateral gaze, sometimes adding up with a horizontal gaze-evoked nystagmus to an oblique pattern. Saccadic pursuit and defective VOR suppression are commonly associated. On Romberg testing, patients tend to sway backwards. Other cerebellar signs are often lacking (video clip 07.04).

The exact mechanism of downbeat nystagmus is unknown. One hypothesis suspects disinhibition of the anterior canal vestibulo-ocular reflex because the caudal cerebellum inhibits signals from the anterior canal more effectively than those from the antagonistic posterior canal. In many patients no definite cause can be found (idiopathic downbeat nystagmus) but one should make sure that cerebellar pathology (Chiari malformation, degenerations, paraneoplastic), and toxicity (carabamazepine, phenytoin, lithium, alcohol) are excluded.

Treatment with 4-aminopyridine may lead to improvement of oscillopsia and mobility, but only rarely to a clinically significant extent. Clonazepam, baclofen and memantine had some effect on nystagmus intensity in several small case series. Operating on a patient with Chiari malformation should be considered when there are troublesome brainstem or cerebellar symptoms, particularly if worsened by Valsalva manoevres.

If the degree of unsteadiness appears excessive to the cerebellar deficit, make sure that your patient does not have additional bilateral vestibulopathy or peripheral neuropathy (the 'CANVAS' syndrome – Cerebellar Atrophy, Neuropathy, Vestibular Areflexia Syndrome). Due to the combination of absent pursuit (cerebellar function) and bilateral vestibular failure these patients show a useful sign during the slow doll's head-eye manoeuvre. Whereas in normal subjects this manoeuvre elicits perfectly smooth eye movements (video clip 02.12) in the CANVAS patient the eye movement is extremely saccadic or 'broken up'.

Parkinsonism and Parkinson's disease

In its early stages Parkinson's disease is difficult to diagnose. Unilateral resting tremor ('pill rolling'), the most distinctive feature of Parkinson's disease, is lacking in more than half of the patients at this time and sometimes for the entire course of the disease. Instead, patients may complain about unsteadiness, loss of dexterity, hoarseness, stiffness, muscle aches and 'lack of energy'. On examination, one can search for hypokinesia by asking the patient to perform rapidly alternating hand movements, to get up from a chair and to turn 360 degrees on the spot, which should take no more than six steps. Unilateral loss of arm swing during walking is another early sign, whereas the characteristic slow, small-stepped and shuffling gait with hesitation and postural instability develops only later on (video clips 07.05 and 07.06). Rigidity is best noted when the patient performs gripping hand movements on one side while the contralateral arm is passively moved by the examiner; asymmetric 'cog wheeling' during this manoeuvre is a useful early sign. Improvement of symptoms after a single dose of 100 or 200 mg L-dopa (after premedication with domperidone to prevent

Video 07.05 – Impaired postural reflexes
The video clip shows a patient who complains of gait unsteadiness. First the Romberg test is performed. Then several short clips are shown when the patient is pushed forward or backwards. Particularly when the trunk is pulled backwards the patient either falls or develops inefficient shuffling backwards steps. This patient has gait ataxia, retropulsion and abnormal postural reflexes as shown and the diagnosis was cerebral small-vessel disease.

Video 07.06 – High level gait disorder (freezing and hesitation)
The video clip shows a patient complaining of dizziness and unsteadiness. She described her episodes of gait hesitation during turning, and partial freezing just before going through the door frame, as dizziness and disorientation. The MRI showed white-matter ischemic features and involutional changes.

Video 07.07 – Early PSP: eyes
Both horizontal and vertical saccades are slow and fragmented in this patient with progressive supranuclear palsy. In addition, there is partial upward gaze palsy which corresponds to a more severe dysfunction of the saccadic system.

Video 07.08 – Early PSP: gait
Gait in early akinetic-rigid syndrome: this patient with a possible diagnosis of progressive supranuclear palsy (PSP) shows a slightly broad-based gait and reduction of walking speed, lack of normal arm swing during walking and slow gait turns.

Video 07.09 – Early PSP: Romberg
Romberg test in a patient with an early akinetic-rigid syndrome: normal levels of postural sway with eyes open and closed. Due to the slight abnormality of gait and postural reactions shown in the accompanying videos, this patient can describe unsteadiness or even dizziness despite the completely normal Romberg test shown in this video shot.

Video 07.10 – Early PSP: postural reflexes
Abnormal postural reactions in a patient with an early akinetic-rigid syndrome: during backwards pulls to the trunk the patient consistently takes two or more protective steps. During forward pushes the patient is slow to use her feet to generate protective steps and often relies on her arms.

nausea) is another diagnostic criterion for Parkinson's disease. If the patient has a prominent tremor, a dopamine transport (DAT) scan will be abnormally positive in Parkinson's disease but normal in essential tremor, a common condition which does not produce significant balance symptoms.

In addition to the typical idiopathic Parkinson's disease described above, there are other (less treatable) parkinsonian syndromes, which can usually be diagnosed by the presence of additional symptoms and signs. Slow saccades (video clip 02.27), vertical gaze limitation and early falls point to progressive supranuclear palsy (video clips 07.05–07.10). Autonomic symptoms (orthostatic hypotension, erectile dysfunction) and cerebellar signs (loss of VOR suppression, positional downbeat nystagmus) suggest multiple system atrophy. The presence of mild dementia, urge incontinence and a compatible MRI scan indicate normal-pressure hydrocephalus or cerebral small-vessel disease. In practice, early falls and lack of response to L-dopa frequently suggest that the patient suffers from parkinsonism rather than Parkinson's disease – examine these patients carefully for confirmatory additional signs as described above.

A diagnosis of Parkinson's disease should not be missed because anti-Parkinson drugs such as L-dopa and dopamine agonists can relieve symptoms by about 70%, even if doses need to be increased in later stages of the disease.

Normal-pressure hydrocephalus

Normal-pressure hydrocephalus is actually a misnomer because the ventricular enlargement in this condition is the consequence of brief and moderate increases in cerebrospinal fluid (CSF) pressure. Clinically, these elderly patients present with a triad of gait disorder, urge incontinence and slight dementia. (Note that the clinical features are quite similar to cerebral small-vessel disease, see page 152.) Abnormal gait is the earliest and most prominent symptom and is characterised by a hesitant, non-fluent cadence, often with some stiffness and a moderately widened base, as well as imbalance on turning around. As the disease progresses the gait becomes increasingly small-stepped and may lead to falls, eventually immobilising the patient. Cranial CT or MRI shows enlarged ventricles while external CSF spaces are normal or even narrowed over the vertex. In addition, there are hypodense (CT) or T2-hyperintense (MRI) white-matter alterations around the anterior and posterior extensions of the lateral ventricles (pressure caps), which result from CSF pressed into the adjacent white matter.

A lumbar puncture with removal of 50 ml CSF produces a substantial gait improvement within a day or two. This can be measured by the time and the number of steps needed to walk a defined distance before and after puncture. This finding further supports the diagnosis but it cannot be claimed to be confirmatory. In equivocal cases, CSF can be drained continuously for three days with an indwelling spinal catheter. Long-term treatment requires CSF drainage through a ventriculo-peritoneal shunt which will also improve cognitive and bladder symptoms. Unfortunately, however, it is not easy to predict which patients will truly benefit from the neurosurgical treatment.

Fear of falling and cautious gait

Fear of falling can develop in fallers (sometimes after just a single fall) and in patients who have sustained a vestibular disorder, but also in elderly patients who have never fallen and look otherwise normal. This can be associated with a 'cautious gait' with reduced stride length and speed or even sliding the feet on the floor as if 'walking on ice'. The arms are outstretched and seeking support. One has to be careful in dismissing these patients' problems as purely psychogenic or functional because a cautious gait sometimes masks an objective gait disorder. It would seem that the patients react to a perceived unsteadiness before it is apparent to an observer. Balance and gait training and confidence building led by an experienced physiotherapist is usually helpful.

Cardiac arrhythmia

Cardiac arrhythmia is a frequent cause of dizziness in the elderly, not only because heart disease is so common in this age group but also because arrhythmia rapidly causes symptomatic cerebral hypoperfusion when cerebral autoregulation is impaired. Concomitant congestive heart failure may further increase the susceptibility to arrhythmia-induced dizziness. Patients with paroxysmal cardiac arrhythmia typically report episodes with light-headedness lasting seconds, which are sometimes accompanied by palpitations and which may evolve to syncope. Further details are discussed in Chapter 4, page 97.

Orthopaedic disorders

Isolated orthopaedic problems cannot explain recurrent or chronic dizziness. However, imbalance may be aggravated by decreased mobility of leg joints and the lumbar spine interfering with rapid postural adjustments. The most common condition is osteoarthritis of the hip before or after surgical replacement. In operated patients, sensory deafferentation of the joint may contribute to the balance problem.

'Cervical vertigo' is a long-lived myth that tries to explain a symptom of the brain by disease of the bone. Most experts in the field agree that the most common cause of 'neck-movement-induced vertigo' is a vestibular disorder, so a Hallpike manoeuvre for detection of BPPV should always be performed in these patients (see Figure 5.1). Migraine headaches involve the neck in about 50% of patients. Therefore, vestibular migraine is a common cause of recurrent vertigo with neck pain. Another consideration is that a primary vestibular disorder often results in stiffening up of the neck – a protective reaction to avoid further dizziness on head movements. Combined neck and vestibular physiotherapy usually breaks up this vicious circle.

Falls in the elderly

The problem of the elderly faller has steadily grown in industrialised societies to the point of being a major public health issue. This is due to two factors. First, life expectancy has increased worldwide; and second, morbidity and mortality associated with falls is high in the elderly. A simple fall is a trivial event in a young, fit person but may cause fractures in the elderly, if there is underlying osteoporosis, and then hospitalisation, with many potential secondary complications, including death.

In order to develop a rational approach to the elderly faller it may be useful to divide the problem into predisposing factors, specific disorders leading to falls, and accompanying symptoms indicating the cause of a fall ('funny turns'). A checklist displayed in the consulting room may help the clinician organise the consultation of this multifactorial problem (Tables 7.3, 7.4 and 7.5).

A general predisposing factor to falls in the elderly is, naturally, the normal, age-related decrement in balance control. Balance is a process dependent on a number of peripheral sensory inputs (chiefly proprioceptive, visual and vestibular) integrated centrally with each other and combined with other relevant neural functions such as motor control and cognition. A vast amount of research has confirmed that the elderly suffer from age-related loss of function in each of these sensory and central processes. Also, correlations exist between simple measured variables (e.g. loss of peripheral input such as proprioception and increase in postural sway) and between more complex measures (e.g. increase in postural sway or decrement in walking speed and falls in everyday life). However, the current view is that normal ageing per se should not be held responsible for falls. This puts clinicians in 'active search mode' – an underlying pathological process or processes should be sought in the elderly faller, in the hope that treatment or preventive measures can be identified.

Cognitive status is an important predictive factor for falls. Dementia cannot produce a fall per se, but two aspects are important. Many dementing processes such as vascular dementia, normal-pressure hydrocephalus and atypical parkinsonian syndromes are associated with gait disorders directly responsible for falls. But even in dementias with relatively little motor disorder, such as Alzheimer's disease, the memory or spatial disorientation

Table 7.3 Essential investigations for falls in the elderly

• History and clinical examination – identify general predisposing factors	Age-related balance dysfunction
	Cognitive problems
	Visual impairment
	'Foot and shoe' disorders
	Dizziness
	Gait unsteadiness
	Psychotropic drugs and polymedication
	Sedentary lifestyle
• Funny turn or loss of consciousness? Consider:	
BP supine and standing	Orthostatic hypotension
24 hour ECG	Cardiac arrhythmia
Hallpike test	BPPV
EEG	Epilepsy
Blood glucose	Hypoglycaemia
• Neurological gait disorder? Consider:	Previous stroke, e.g. hemiparesis
General neurological, gait and eye-movement examination, brain and spine imaging	Ischaemic white-matter disease
	Hydrocephalus
	Parkinsonian syndrome
	Cerebellar disease
	Cervical myelopathy
	Peripheral neuropathy (e.g. alcohol, diabetic)

BP = blood pressure; ECG = electrocardiogram; EEG = electroencephalogram; BPPV = benign paroxysmal positional vertigo

disorder, lack of insight or poor 'risk assessment' conducted by the patients in unexpected situations may put them in hazardous situations.

Psychotropic drugs, in particular polypharmacy, have been repeatedly identified as an important contributory factor to falls in the elderly. One should ask the patient, the referring doctor and indeed oneself, whether all the medications that the patient is taking are really necessary. In the specific case of hypnotics, are there any lifestyle measures that the patient could adopt to improve sleep, such as avoiding daytime naps, increasing physical activity during the day and cutting down alcohol and caffeine in the evening?

Vision and the patient's environment are interrelated. Many falls are triggered by tripping over. If vision is poor the patient, naturally, does not see the obstacle. However, even patients with good vision trip over and fall because of poorly lit rooms, loose rugs, low coffee tables and wires, heaters or fans on the floor. A visit to the optician, or if required a referral to the ophthalmologist, may be indicated. Similarly, a visit by a nurse, occupational therapist, or an intelligent family member instructed to search the patient's house for potential foot obstacles, may be of help.

Leg and foot disorders, particularly painful arthritic conditions, contribute to falls. These disorders lead to inactivity and secondary weakness by disuse. In addition, important rescue postural reactions needed to avoid a fall may be impossible due to pain and limited motion range. Always enquire about pain and limitations in the leg and examine

Table 7.4 Specific disorders leading to falls

Stroke sequelae (e.g. hemiparesis)

Small-vessel white-matter disease (leucoaraiosis)

Hydrocephalus

Parkinsonian syndromes

Higher-order disorders (e.g. frontal gait ignition failure)

Cerebellar disease (e.g. the downbeat nystagmus syndrome)

Cervical spondylogenic myelopathy

Peripheral neuropathy

Table 7.5 'Funny turns': additional neurological symptoms as a clue to causes of falls

Symptoms	Disorder
Blackening out of vision, light-headedness, loss of consciousness (LOC)	Syncope, due to orthostatic hypotension cardio- or neurally mediated (vasovagal, micturition, cough)
Déjà vu, epigastric or other aura, focal myoclonus, automatisms	Epilepsy
Brief vertigo after neck extension or bending forward	Benign paroxysmal positional vertigo
Clouding of consciousness, hunger, unusual behaviour	Hypoglycaemia

accordingly. Anti-inflammatory/analgesic drugs or a referral to the orthopaedic surgeon may be needed. Remember to examine the patient's legs and gait but also his/her footwear. Inappropriate shoes do contribute to trips, falls and fractures. Shoes that are too flexible and give no support – typically slippers that the elderly are so fond of – are particularly risky.

Dizziness is associated with falls but there are at least three mechanisms linking the two symptoms. 'Proper' vestibular dizziness, say vertigo due to BPPV in an old lady hanging clothes on the washing line, may cause a fall. More frequently the patient reports either vague episodic dizziness, as in presyncopal situations (see below), or a continuous sensation of feeling off-balance, as in disequilibrium due to sensorimotor neurological disorders (Tables 6.2 and 7.4).

Specific factors inducing falls

The specific neurologic disorders leading to falls are identical to those causing imbalance (Table 7.4; for details see page 153).

Loss of consciousness

A key question to answer in anybody who suffers from falls is whether or not there has been loss of consciousness (LOC). This information can come from the patient or a reliable witness. If one could ascertain the answer reliably, half of the job would be done:

if there is LOC it is likely to be syncope (cardiogenic or neurogenic), epilepsy or hypoglycaemia; if there isn't then it is likely to be a balance or gait disorder. Unfortunately, determining the presence of LOC in the elderly is not as easy as it seems. Many patients cannot be sure whether there has been LOC or not, they just find themselves on the floor. Sometimes the LOC is just trivialised ('Maybe I was out but just for a couple of seconds') or not remembered at all. Even in the cognitively normal elderly person there is retrograde amnesia for independently confirmed syncopal LOC in up to 30% of cases (Table 7.5).

Syncope

It can be difficult to diagnose a fall due to a loss of consciousness and the list of possible diagnoses is long. One should at least ask these questions: is it syncope (neurogenic or cardiogenic)? Is it epilepsy? Is it a metabolic disorder (e.g. hypoglycaemia)? Although BPPV does not cause LOC, for the reasons mentioned above (poor memory in many patients), BPPV and other paroxysmal vestibular disorders are often included in the differential diagnosis. Hypoglycaemia is usually clear from the history but blood sugar levels should be monitored nevertheless.

The more common cause of falls due to LOC is syncope, defined as a transient loss of consciousness due to an abrupt decrease in cerebral blood flow. Before losing consciousness and falling, patients often report dizziness, blurred vision, pressured or blocked ears or tinnitus, feeling hot or cold with a clammy sweat. Witnesses say that patients usually look pale. Those with cardiogenic syncope may report palpitations or chest pain. Patients with syncope often suffer 'presyncopal' episodes in which they just report dizziness or light-headedness. However, syncope is an umbrella syndrome with the more common types in the elderly being orthostatic hypotension, neurally mediated (vasovagal) syncope and cardiac arrhythmias. Although we will not discuss cardiogenic syncope here, the clinician should know that a cardiological opinion is often useful and mandatory in the patient with unexplained LOC or chest symptoms. Unlike neurogenic syncope, cardiogenic syncope is the one that can kill your patient. On a positive note, a good cardiologist and a pacemaker often get rid of unexplained episodes of dizziness or falls.

Orthostatic hypotension

Patients with dizziness and falls related to postural hypotension describe their dizziness as light-headedness but 'true' vertigo can be reported as well. Patients are often aware of the need to lie/sit down. Falls occurring immediately after standing up are suggestive. More details on orthostatic hypotension, including postprandial hypotension, are given on page 94.

Neurally mediated syncope

Neurogenic syncope, as the name indicates, involves bradycardia and/or hypotension brought about by an autonomic reflex mechanism. The main types are vasovagal syncope ('common faints') and situational syncope (e.g. during coughing or urinating), while syncope due to carotid sinus hypersensitivity seems to be rare. Patients with vasovagal episodes may have a previous lifelong history of faints and know how to prevent them by sitting or lying down. Vasovagal episodes have clear precipitating events (fear, pain or emotions, such as the sight of blood) and relatively long prodromes, such as feeling hot and bothered in a stuffy room particularly in prolonged periods of standing. In contrast, the carotid sinus syndrome induces typically sudden and unpredictable syncope, often in connection with mechanical stimuli to the neck such as shaving or tie knotting. However, isolated laboratory evidence of carotid sinus hypersensitivity, in the absence of a typical history and exclusion of other causes of falls or syncope, should be taken with caution as an explanation for the patient's falls. For proof of carotid sinus hypersensitivity an ECG needs to be recorded during the individual provoking activity.

Epilepsy

The paroxysmal neurological disorders that should be taken into consideration if a 'funny turn' is thought to be the cause of a fall are epilepsy and BPPV. In contrast, cerebrovascular episodes (TIAs) show focal neurological symptoms such as hemiparesis/hemianaesthesia, double vision and speech disturbance but loss of consciousness is rare. Epilepsy is common in the elderly because the incidence of this condition follows a bi-modal distribution, with one peak in childhood and a second in old age. This is due to the age-related increase in diseases capable of producing seizures, particularly cerebrovascular disease, but also tumours, head injury, subdural haematoma and mixed causes.

Owing to the prevalence of structural causes in the elderly, partial (i.e. focal) epilepsy is more common than idiopathic generalised epilepsy. Patients with unilateral limb seizures, with or without secondary weakness, may be wrongly diagnosed as having TIA. Indications that the patient with loss of consciousness suffers from epilepsy may come from reliable witnesses, in particular the observation of stereotyped fits. Persistent confusion or head-aches after an episode of loss of consciousness are suggestive of epilepsy.

Any patient with focal neurological symptoms or signs, and any patient who develops epilepsy, with or without focal signs, should have a CT or MRI scan. An EEG may be required for classifying the type of epilepsy (i.e. partial or generalised). However, since the diagnosis of epilepsy is clinical, a normal EEG does not mean that the patient does not have epilepsy, nor should one withhold treatment in somebody with unequivocal fits. In some cases, a therapeutic trial with an antiepileptic drug such as lamotrigine or levetiracetam may be justified.

Drop attacks

This diagnosis implies that the patient 'just drops', buckling at the knees without warning, clouding of consciousness, additional symptoms or postictal phenomena. Patients may just get up and carry on walking. In those with repeated drop attacks the knees appear bruised and scarred. Explanations based on a transient brainstem ischaemia apply only to a minority of mostly elderly patients with vascular risk factors. Superior cerebellar artery occlusion starts with a sudden fall in 50% of patients, indicating that posterior fossa ischaemia may indeed lead to drop attacks. However, the vascular hypothesis is unconvincing for most of these patients, who do not show a particularly high cerebrovascular risk and do not have associated brainstem symptoms. In contrast, the largest subgroups are young and middle-aged women who are otherwise healthy (so-called *idiopathic drop attacks*). The French term *la maladie des genoux bleus* highlights the risk for injuries including fractures. Another complication is secondary agoraphobia which may require specific therapy. An effective treatment for prevention of idiopathic drop attacks has not been established.

A specific type of drop attacks occurs in some patients with Ménière's disease, so-called *Tumarkin attacks*, which are perceived by patients as if being pushed to the ground by an external force. These attacks probably reflect unstable otolithic function. Patients usually have few attacks stretched over several weeks or months before spontaneous remission occurs. Persistent attacks can be treated by transtympanic injections of steroids or gentamicin into the affected ear (see page 83). Drop attacks occur also with non-Ménière vestibulopathies including superior canal dehiscence and vestibular paroxysmia and with presyncope, Chiari malformation and spinal ischaemia. The differential diagnosis includes falls due to cataplexy caused by a sudden loss of muscle tone triggered by sudden emotions. They are part of the narcolepsy – cataplexy syndrome which causes daytime sleepiness as a principal symptom. In vestibular falls there is usually a component of sideways push or lateropulsion rather than truly buckling at the knees.

The concept of drop attacks can have a negative impact on the investigation of a patient with falls. It often provides an escape route for the doctor rather than encouraging him/her to pursue an intelligent investigation of the problem. Always enquire about features suggestive of syncope, paroxysmal vestibular disorder or brainstem TIA, and examine the patient to make sure there is no neurological disorder of balance and gait.

Approach to the patient with falls

Patients should have a thorough assessment, because even when there is an apparently obvious cause for a fall – say, advanced Parkinson's disease – many additional factors may be playing a significant part as well. Attention should be given to the medications received, such as antihypertensive and anti-prostate hypoplasia agents (orthostatic hypotension?), hypoglycaemic agents and psychotropic drugs.

From the history, try to establish what the patient was doing at the time of the fall (had just stood up, walking, standing quietly, looking up?). Try to identify: (a) whether there was loss of consciousness; and (b) the events immediately preceding the fall, such as presyncopal features, sudden standing up, coughing, micturition, neck turns (BPPV, carotid syndrome?), palpitations, focal fits, tripping over, or 'freezing' of the legs on turning (parkinsonian and gait apraxic syndromes?, video clips 07.05–07.10).

The examinations likely to be the focus of attention are cardiovascular, neurological and a positional manoeuvre. Also obtain general blood tests for metabolic disorders such as hypoglycaemia. Remember to look at the feet and shoes.

A cardiovascular examination should be carried out in all cases, including routine ECG and blood pressure in the supine and orthostatic positions for up to three minutes. Special investigations such as prolonged combined ambulatory ECG and blood pressure monitoring as well as tilt-table should be considered when there have been recurrent unexplained falls. You should know that this is what your faller needs rather than a routine consultation with a cardiologist who might examine your patient only in the supine position.

In your neurological assessment, observe the patient's stance with eyes open and closed. How does he walk (straight and on turning)? Can she walk in tandem (heel-to-toe)? How does he react to trunk pushes and pulls (push but be ready to catch!– see video clips 07.05 and 07.10)? Can she sit and stand up without difficulty? Does she rely heavily on her arms for this task? Unless pain or orthopaedic disability is present, any abnormality noted during this global assessment is likely to indicate an underlying neurological disorder of gait or balance. Further clinical neurological examination is then warranted; either proceed yourself or refer to a neurologist. EEG (epilepsy?) or brain scan (space-occupying lesion, vascular disease, hydrocephalus?) may be required.

Management of the faller

From the history and examinations outlined in the previous sections, many conditions that respond to specific measures are likely to be found. Examples are adjustments in antidiabetic, antihypertensive, alpha blockers (prostate) and hypnotic medications, pacemaker implantation, antiepileptic medication, or a repositioning procedure for BPPV. That said, you will be left with many patients in whom no definite cause can be found and the problem is then multifactorial.

There is some evidence that a home assessment can help to prevent falls. There is more solid evidence that exercise regimens to promote leg strengthening and balance rehabilitation are effective. For the individual patient one can recommend this without hesitation; however, at a public health level, efforts are being made to target the more vulnerable groups at risk of falling, such as those over 70 years of age with a history of two or more falls or with balance and gait difficulties. Be aware that only active interventions seem to work; education alone is not enough in the elderly: development of a secondary 'fear of falling' syndrome, with the consequent restriction in levels of activity, may lead to a vicious circle. There is no accepted treatment for this syndrome, but combinations of physiotherapy, confidence-building and fitness retraining, often in group sessions, can be effective.

What to do if you don't have a clue

An elderly patient with dizziness or falls can be a real challenge. History-taking is often cumbersome because of multiple problems and poor memory. The physical examination may take time when concentration and mobility are reduced. Eventually, one may end up with various abnormalities but no definite diagnosis. The following points should offer some guidance in this situation.

Take multimorbidity into account

Several minor findings may add up to explain a major balance problem. Also, there may be separate problems, which are all lumped together as 'dizziness' by the patient. Therefore, don't stop too early! For example, it can be useful to do a Hallpike manoeuvre and measure orthostatic blood pressure even after another explanation has been found for the patient's imbalance.

Check somatosensory and motor functions that contribute to balance

The routine vestibular examination is usually not adequate for sorting out a balance problem in the elderly. A complete neurological examination may be required to detect disorders such as peripheral neuropathy, early Parkinson's disease or cerebellar disease (see pages 153–158).

Do not overlook psychiatric aspects

Emotions are alive in the elderly! Balance problems may cause disproportionate disability when secondary anxiety triggers a vicious cycle of avoidance, immobility and decreasing fitness leading to even more anxiety. Depression is another prevalent condition in the elderly and may manifest itself with somatic complaints such as persistent dizziness, headache or fatigue (see page 139).

Request a good cardiological opinion

Paroxysmal cardiac arrhythmias can be life-threatening, explain your patient's symptoms and be easily, at the same time, treated. Chest symptoms may be absent. On a different note, a single normal orthostatic BP measurement does not rule out postural hypotension. Repeat the measurements or refer for autonomic testing.

Remember what elderly patients are *not* likely to have

Old patients may suffer from almost anything but some disorders are rather unlikely to *begin* beyond 70 years of age, including Ménière's disease, vestibular migraine, autoimmune disorders of the inner ear and episodic ataxias. Note, however, that all these disorders may *persist* into old age.

Seek cooperation with specialists in geriatric rehabilitation

This may help to identify functional limitations that can be improved by customised exercises.

Treatment of the dizzy patient

Co-authored with Marousa Pavlou, PhD, physiotherapist,
King's College, London

There are four components to the treatment of a patient with dizziness or vertigo:

- treatment of the specific condition, such as benign paroxysmal positional vertigo (BPPV) or migraine, to name two of the more common ones;
- counselling and reassurance;
- rehabilitation;
- pharmacological treatment of vertigo and associated nausea.

These four aspects should be considered for each individual patient and they are all equally important (Table 8.1). However, not all patients will require action in all four domains. For instance, patients with BPPV will usually require repositioning treatment and nothing else.

Table 8.1 Key elements in the treatment of dizzy patients

• Specific treatment of the underlying condition	Examples: Positional manoeuvres for BPPV Migraine prophylaxis for vestibular migraine Gentamicin for Ménière's disease Antiplatelet agents for TIAs Cognitive behavioural therapy for anxiety disorders
• Reassurance, information, counselling	Relieves unnecessary fears; provides the basis for therapeutic cooperation and realistic goals
• Vestibular rehabilitation	For treatment of chronic dizziness and imbalance. Includes exercises for: Eye–head coordination Retraining of balance strategies Gait training Visual desensitisation Ball games
• Non-specific drug treatment of acute vertigo, nausea and vomiting	For example: dimenhydrinate, prochlorperazine, promethazine
• Other treatments	Surgery (e.g. refractory BPPV, Ménière's) Stress management Self-help groups

BPPV = benign paroxysmal positional vertigo
TIA = transient ischaemic attack

Patients with chronic dizziness usually require counselling and rehabilitation but no drugs. In contrast, patients with vestibular migraine, if they do not have interictal symptoms, may just require antimigraine drugs but no rehabilitation. As always in medicine, the treatment has to be tailored to the individual patient.

Patient reassurance, information and counselling

Vertigo is a terrifying experience, particularly the very first attack. Most patients associate the sensation with life-threatening or incapacitating conditions such as a heart attack, stroke or even imminent death. Patients with conditions such as BPPV or vestibular neuritis need to be reassured that, despite the unpleasant symptoms they experience, the underlying cause is benign. In our experience patients also need an explanation as to why they feel they are spinning around, and this can be achieved with simple drawings of the semicircular canals and a comment on their normal function in sensing head rotation. Other patients, on learning that the problem is in the inner ear, worry about the possibility of going deaf. In the more common conditions such as migraine, BPPV or vestibular neuritis, reassurance in this regard can be provided. An audiogram can be useful to confirm normal hearing or that the patient's hearing problem may be unrelated (e.g. presbyacusis or middle-ear dysfunction).

The patient with acute vertigo also needs a brief explanation on the process of vestibular compensation. Typically, when patients learn that 'the balance organs of the inner ear on one side are damaged' they want to know whether 'what has been lost will ever grow back'. At this point reassurance on the power of the brain to make up for the loss of peripheral function is needed. This is also a good opportunity to explain that rest, in particular bed-rest, is *not* indicated – quite the contrary. They should understand that for the process of vestibular compensation to be successful they should try to remain active and limit activity moderately only during the hyperacute phase. However, 'too keen' patients should also be told not to overdo it, because of the possibility that nausea or vomiting could lead to exhaustion and future negative associations between physical activity and nausea (a kind of 'conditioned response' of the type experienced by some people who think of a boat in rough seas and can actually feel sick).

Patients with long-term dizziness need quite a lot of reassurance. These patients have often wandered from clinic to clinic, from specialist to specialist, sometimes for months or years. On the basis of normal brain scans some doctor is likely to have said, at some point, 'there's nothing wrong with you', or 'there's nothing that medical science can do for you', or 'it's all in your mind'. We believe that this is not only the wrong approach but also usually not true. Patients may have suffered a genuine vestibular insult in the past, which may not show in conventional vestibular testing, but failures in the vestibular compensation process or secondary added psychological problems complicate the situation. It is a fact that rehabilitation works even in patients with many years of chronic dizzy symptoms, so you want your patient to cooperate in this process. For this reason you need to explain the principles of vestibular compensation and rehabilitation. You may also need to mention that symptoms of anxiety and depression are very common in patients with dizziness – but that this doesn't imply that the symptoms are imaginary or, worse, the result of malingering.

In departments seeing large numbers of patients with dizziness and vertigo it is customary to have leaflets with patient-oriented information. Many of these are available from websites, such as the British Brain and Spine Foundation (www.bbsf.org.uk), the Ménière's Society (www.menieres.org.uk) or the Vestibular Disorders Association (www.vestibular.org) (see page 184, Media for patients). Apart from the factual information they provide, leaflets reassure patients because they can see their symptoms and problems described, and solutions to these presented – light at the end of the tunnel. Self-help groups, in which patients share information and experiences, can be similarly effective. In these days of Internet-acquired knowledge most patients or their relatives will be able to obtain information on local groups working on dizziness, tinnitus, falls, migraine or stress management. Most doctors, therapists or social services should have local knowledge and recommend specialised charities or patient-based groups capable of providing additional help.

Rehabilitation

A key aspect in rehabilitation of balance disorders is the understanding that control of balance emerges from an interaction between many sensorimotor systems. The purpose of rehabilitation is to facilitate the ability of the central nervous system (CNS) to compensate for lesions in the vestibular system. The neural basis for vestibular compensation is distributed throughout the nervous system such that lesions in the cerebellum, cortex, spinal cord, brainstem or sensory systems can prevent or reduce the capacity for compensation. As mentioned in Chapter 2, vestibular compensation is a plastic process that allows the CNS to redress functional symmetry after a unilateral peripheral vestibular lesion. Patients with both unilateral and bilateral vestibular loss also compensate by a process of sensory substitution. In both cases, but particularly the latter, patients learn to rely more on non-vestibular information for balance, namely visual and proprioceptive inputs. Although this is obviously a useful compensatory process, we will see later on that it can also create some new problems (e.g. visual vertigo, page 134).

In this section we will discuss the general principles and techniques employed in the rehabilitation of vestibular patients. We aim to outline how to organise a rehabilitation programme for a dizzy patient because we know that many doctors may not have access to an audiologist or physiotherapist specifically trained in vestibular rehabilitation. However, this is not ideal and, in the long run, you will need access to a trained therapist.

Rehabilitation assessment

In order to rehabilitate vestibular patients, a thorough balance and vertigo assessment is required (Table 8.2). Medical practitioners should understand that what matters now are *symptoms, (dys)function and activity limitation* per se – not an aetiological diagnosis. In addition, many patients with vestibular pathology develop secondary problems, including musculoskeletal impairments resulting from increased muscle tension, stress or fatigue. These secondary problems can affect both functional mobility skills and the patient's ability to effectively participate in a rehabilitation programme. Inactivity, whether from bed-rest, fear, anxiety or other factors, also delays and impairs complete compensation. Other factors that can affect the capacity to compensate for a vestibular lesion are listed in Table 8.3. Every effort should be made to identify and act on each of these negative components, from analgesic drugs or referral to a musculoskeletal physiotherapist for a painful neck or hip, to psychological counselling if indicated.

Table 8.2 Essentials of rehabilitation assessment

Functional assessment	Standard: Romberg, tandem gait Specific: 'get up and go test', timed gait
Symptom assessment	Triggers: e.g. head or visual movement Limitations to treatment: e.g. cervical pain
System assessment	Musculoskeletal: flexibility and range of motion Neuromuscular: power and coordination Sensory: sensory systems and 'weighting'

Table 8.3 Factors interfering with clinical recovery following vestibular lesions

Age

Lesions in the central nervous system

Peripheral somatosensory disorders

Visual disorders:
  reduced visual acuity
  modified optics (e.g. cataract operation)
  strabismus

Visual dependence

Cervical or other spine disorders

Psycho-social problems

Medical treatment:
  surgical procedures
  antivertiginous drugs
  tranquillisers
  anaesthesia

Lack of mobility:
  orthopaedic (e.g. hip arthritis)
  excessive bed-rest or patient advised not to move
  psychological/fear

Functional assessment

The functional assessment is partly incorporated into the clinical examination such as the Romberg test and gait assessment including tandem or heel-to-toes gait. In addition, observing the patient through sequential actions which can be rated or timed may be useful. For example, the 'Get up and go' test is a quick screening tool for detecting balance problems in the elderly. This examination allows a clinician to determine the level of performance of functional tasks of balance in the patient with a peripheral or central neural lesion. They are useful for evaluating the effectiveness of therapy but do not provide insight into the underlying sensory and motor impairments of individual systems.

Systems assessment

The systems assessment partly implies detecting additional sensorimotor or musculoskeletal disorders that vestibular patients might have. Somatosensory, visual and motor function can be examined with a conventional neurological examination. However, even when each individual sensory system is functioning normally, the type and degree of sensory information used to control postural balance varies from subject to subject. For instance, 'visually dependent' patients report dizziness symptoms in visually challenging situations (crowds, driving, supermarkets, looking at moving visual scenes). Visual dependence can be identified in the laboratory or by a specialised physiotherapist, but a few questions identifying visual triggers may suffice (see later).

Symptom assessment

Symptom assessment involves identifying the primary vestibular symptom and its associated autonomic and psychological features. The latter in particular may require additional reassurance or treatment if the patient develops anxiety or hyperventilation.

Identification of triggers

It is most important to identify the presence of triggers for the dizziness (e.g. visual, positional) as this should guide the therapy directly. Some of the common triggers and ways of probing them are described below. Since the principle is 'we'll work on whatever turns your dizziness on' (i.e. desensitisation treatment), the exercises for the patient will largely be based on the findings here.

- *Eye movements.* Patients should do repetitive convergence, pursuit and saccadic eye movements in all directions.
- *Head movements.* Oscillate the head horizontally, vertically and in roll (right ear to right shoulder and left ear to left shoulder).
- *Combined head–eye movements* (horizontally and vertically):
  - *Gaze transference.* Fast eye–head movements are used to refixate objects at 90–180 degrees apart (e.g. lamp in the ceiling to your shoes, and vice versa).
  - *Gaze stability.* Patient keeps the eyes fixed on a stationary object whilst oscillating the head (horizontal and vertical) – essentially VOR excercises.
  - *Gaze or visuo-vestibular conflict.* Patient holds thumbs up or a magazine at arms length and attempts to read whilst oscillating 'en bloc' (head, body and arms together) – essentially VOR suppression excercises.
- *Positional triggers.* If there is BPPV this should have already been treated with repositioning procedures (see Chapter 5, Figures. 5.3, 5.4 and 5.5). However, all vestibular patients, and those who had BPPV in particular, can experience symptoms or be reluctant to lie down fully and roll over in bed; similarly with bending over and looking up (as when looking for something on a high shelf). These potential triggers should be interrogated *and* examined.
- *Environmental triggers.*
  - *Visual triggers.* Simple questions are sufficient to identify visually aggravated dizziness ('visual vertigo', page 134), such as discomfort when viewing moving

scenes or projections, movements of crowds or traffic, busy supermarkets, movement of curtains, ironing striped shirts, movement of clouds or foliage. Some of these patients are 'visually dependent'; that is, they are using vision too much to compensate for their vestibular problem. The problem is that visual information, as in some of the examples provided, can be unstable and misleading, hence leading to dizziness.

– *Proprioceptive or 'surface' triggers*. These can be assessed by balancing on an unstable surface ('wobbleboard'), balancing and walking on compliant surfaces (mattress, rubber foam) and walking up/down ramps. Balance and gait with eyes closed should also be examined.

Rehabilitation of balance disorders

Vestibular exercises (video clips 08.01 and 08.02)

Essentially these consist of eye, head and postural exercises of progressive complexity (Table 8.4). The exercises the patient is asked to perform are intended to include the eye, head or body positions and movements that provoke vertigo. Since the aim is to stimulate the vestibular system, patients should come off medication as early as possible. However, medication can be used to suppress symptoms during the early stages of therapy.

The exercises should be performed for 10–15 minutes twice a day. Pacing of the exercises is crucial. Unless they are performed slowly at first they will induce an unacceptable degree of vertigo and nausea. However, the patient should be instructed to gradually increase the pace and difficulty of the exercises as the provoked vertigo progressively abates. It is important to foster positive but realistic expectations. Patients must be told that their symptoms will at first worsen, and that improvement may be uneven. Clinical trials of the efficacy of exercise programmes typically report improvement in symptoms in 70–80% of those participating. Although generic exercise programmes, either as leaflets or as group physiotherapy sessions, achieve good results, customised therapy results are superior.

Retraining sensory and movement strategies

Some patients, particularly the elderly or those with a CNS disorder, may need additional instruction for developing appropriate postural responses. Patients must practise movement strategies that are successful in controlling the centre of mass relative to the base of support, including: (a) strategies that move the centre of mass relative to a stationary base of support (e.g. an ankle or hip strategy), and (b) strategies for changing the base of support when the centre of mass moves beyond it (e.g. a stepping strategy).

Video 08.01 – Vestibular rehabilitation: seated exercises

The video clip shows some of the head, eye and head–eye exercises appropriate for the rehabilitation of patients with peripheral vestibular disorders.

Video 08.02 – Vestibular rehabilitation: standing exercises

This video clip shows further vestibular exercises, now in the more challenging upright position and then while walking.

Table 8.4 Movements typically included in vestibular rehabilitation programmes (video clips 08.01 and 08.02)

Head exercises (performed with eyes open and closed)

Bend head backwards and forwards

Turn head from side to side

Tilt head from one shoulder to the other

Fixation exercises

Move eyes up and down, side-to-side

Perform head exercises while fixating stationary target

Perform head exercises while fixating moving target

Positioning exercises (performed with eyes open and closed)

While seated, bend down to touch the floor

Bend down with head twisted first to one side and then the other

Lying down, roll from one side to the other

Sit up from lying on the back and on each side

Repeat with head turned to each side

Postural exercises (performed with eyes open; eyes closed under supervision)

Practise static stance with feet as close together as possible

Practise standing on one leg, and heel-to-toe

Repeat head and fixation exercises while standing and then walking

Practise walking in circles, pivot turns, up slopes, stairs, around obstacles

Standing and walking in environments with altered surface and/or visual conditions with and without head and fixation exercises

Aerobic exercises including alternative touching the fingers to the toes, trunk bends and twists, etc.

Developing a coordinated ankle strategy

Patients are asked to practise swaying back and forth, and side to side, within small ranges, keeping the body straight and not bending at the hips or knees. Patients who are very unsteady, or fearful, can practise movement between the parallel bars, standing close to a wall or in a corner with a chair or table in front of them. Use of perturbations applied at the hips or shoulders is an effective way to help patients develop strategies for recovery of balance. Small perturbations are used to facilitate the use of an ankle strategy for balance control. Finally, patients are asked to carry out a variety of manipulation tasks, such as reaching, lifting and throwing, which help them to develop strategies for anticipatory postural control.

Developing a coordinated hip strategy

Larger perturbations, or standing on a narrow beam or in the tandem position, or on a single leg, encourage the use of a hip strategy.

Developing a coordinated step strategy

Learning to step when the centre of mass exceeds the base of support (e.g. as observed during clinical examination of postural responses, see page 44) is an essential part of balance retraining. Initially, stepping can be done within the parallel bars or near a wall or couch in response to pushes or pulls to the shoulders.

Improving orientation and perception

Treatment strategies require the patient to maintain balance during progressively more difficult static and dynamic tasks while the physiotherapist systematically varies the availability and accuracy of sources of information for orientation. Patients with increased reliance on the supporting surface are asked to perform tasks while sitting or standing on surfaces providing decreased somatosensory cues for orientation (foam, tilt or wobble board). Patients who show increased reliance on vision are asked to perform a variety of balance tasks when visual cues are absent (eyes closed or blindfolded), or reduced (diminished lighting). In addition, visual cues can be made inaccurate for orientation through the use of glasses smeared with petroleum jelly, prism glasses, wearing a visual stabilisation dome (e.g. with the head inside a Chinese lantern), or viewing a complex moving visual scene. Finally, in order to enhance the patient's ability to use remaining vestibular information, exercises are given that ask the patient to balance while both visual and somatosensory inputs are simultaneously reduced (e.g. standing on compliant foam or an inclining surface with eyes closed or while wearing petroleum jellied glasses).

Visual desensitisation

In patients reporting enhanced sensitivity or poor tolerance to self or visual motion, additional desensitisation strategies may be added. Decreasing a patient's hypersensitivity to visual motion cues can be done by gradual exposure to optokinetic stimuli, head-mounted video systems or virtual reality sets. A good alternative is to watch computer games or busy video clips (e.g.: Walking through crowds http://www.youtube.com/watch?v=ezyrSKgcyJw; Supermarket http://www.youtube.com/watch?v=bZ4AACQIjul; Escalators https://www.youtube.com/watch?v=XLsgH3nz2EY; Car with windscreen wipers http://www.youtube.com/watch?v=gz-n3I9qd-M; Driving through tunnel http://www.youtube.com/watch?v=AtndQTKH2WE&feature=related). Patients should start in seated conditions and gradually move up to standing, balancing and walking conditions. Side-to-side oscillation, or continuous rotation and stopping, on an office swivel chair with eyes open, closed or in visuovestibular conflict mode (i.e. with a head-fitted Chinese lantern or whilst reading a book) can be easily implemented without resorting to complex rotational equipment. Visual and vestibular stimuli should also start slowly and gradually speed up according to patient tolerance.

Progression

We have tried to outline a comprehensive assessment and rehabilitation plan for vestibular patients, but be reassured that not all patients need so much work-up. In many intelligent and cooperative patients an explanation of the principles of vestibular compensation, and how this is achieved through graded activity, is enough. The next step up would be a list of the exercises, such as in Table 8.4, with an explanation to identify the symptom-provoking exercises, a twice-a-day activity schedule and an indication to intensify the pace progressively. However, try to encourage an audiologist or physiotherapist in your hospital to become

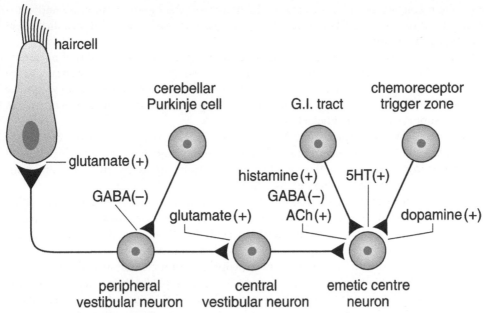

Figure 8.1 **Major neurotransmitters involved in vertigo and emesis.** Note that afferent input to the emetic centre is not necessarily monosynaptic as depicted here for simplicity. ACh = acetylcholine, GABA = γ-aminobutyric acid, 5-HT = 5-hydroxytryptamine (serotonin).

interested in balance rehabilitation. In fact, it has been demonstrated that a general practice nurse can make a very significant difference to the outcome of dizzy patients in primary care.

Drug treatment of vertigo, nausea and vomiting

Pharmacological treatment of vertigo is mostly symptomatic since no drug has been shown to influence a vestibular disorder at the causal level. Two classes of drugs are used for acute vertigo: vestibular suppressants and antiemetics. In the following, we will briefly discuss basic principles of action and indications, before dealing with individual drugs that are commonly used for treatment of vertigo and vomiting. Drug treatment of several specific disorders is discussed elsewhere: for vestibular migraine see Table 4.6, page 78, and for Ménière's disease see page 83.

Mechanisms of action

Although the neurochemistry of the vestibular system has not been fully elucidated, some general principles may help to understand how vestibular suppressants and antiemetics work (Figure 8.1).

Glutamate is the major excitatory transmitter of the vestibular system. Antiglutamatergic drugs are currently not available for treatment of vertigo because glutamate receptors are so widespread within the brain that selective modulation of the vestibular system is hardly possible and disproportionate adverse effects would be inevitable.

Acetylcholine is another excitatory transmitter at the level of the vestibular nuclei. It is also involved in relaying vestibular input to the so-called emetic centre, a group of neurons within the medullary reticular formation which controls the motor, respiratory and autonomic actions of vomiting. Therefore, anticholinergics (e.g. scopolamine) have a dual effect on vertigo and vomiting.

Histamine is widely distributed in central vestibular structures. The action of histamine is complex because various receptor subtypes exist; but the main effect appears to be excitation of neurons in the vestibular nuclei. Moreover, histamine contributes to vestibular activation of the emetic centre. Antihistaminics (e.g. meclizine, cyclizine) are used as vestibular suppressants and antiemetics.

Serotonin (5-hydroxytryptamine, 5-HT) serves to transmit vagal signals from the gastrointestinal tract to the emetic centre. In addition, serotonin modulates the activity of central vestibular neurons. Serotonin antagonists (e.g. ondansetron) suppress mainly vomiting from gastrointestinal causes and chemotherapy which is also relayed by vagal afferents.

Dopamine activates the chemoreceptor trigger zone, an area in the dorsal medulla with a leaky blood–brain barrier that is sensitive to the emetic action of various drugs and toxins. Antidopaminergics (e.g. metoclopramide) have central antiemetic and peripheral gastrokinetic effects, but they do not suppress vertigo and motion sickness.

Gamma-aminobutyric acid (GABA) is the principal inhibitory transmitter of the vestibular system. Cerebellar inhibition of the vestibular nuclei relies on GABAergic neurons. Similarly, vestibular effects on the emetic centre are reduced by GABAergic inhibition. Therefore, GABA agonists (e.g. diazepam) have both vestibular suppressant and antiemetic properties.

Cannabinoids and *neurokinin antagonists* have recently been identified as potent antiemetics but their site of action is less well understood.

How to use vestibular suppressants and antiemetics

The choice of a vestibular suppressant depends on the clinical situation and expected side-effects of the drug (Table 8.5). In particular, potency and sedating effects of vestibular suppressants are closely related. Thus, for patients with acute vertigo, nausea and vomiting, the combination of strong vestibular suppression and sedation can be desirable. Typical disorders would be intense motion sickness, acute vestibular neuritis or severe attacks of Ménière's disease or vestibular migraine. On the other hand, a patient with mild or moderate attacks may get along with a less potent and less sedating drug that allows him or her to continue daily activities. Because the onset of action takes at least 30 minutes and the maximum effect is reached only after one or several hours, brief attacks cannot be treated in this way. Intravenous administration (e.g. diazepam, lorazepam, promethazine) or rectal administration (dimenhydrinate, promethazine, diazepam) can help to shorten the latency between drug intake and effect, and bypass the nauseous stomach.

As a last resort, one may use vestibular suppressants for prophylaxis of recurrent vertigo of unknown cause, which may ameliorate rather than completely eliminate future attacks. When this approach is taken, a less sedating substance should be chosen. For alternative strategies in patients with recurrent vertigo, see page 178.

Often, vestibular suppressants are erroneously prescribed for disorders they cannot control, such as benign paroxysmal positional vertigo, bilateral vestibular loss, poorly compensated unilateral vestibular loss, or chronic dizziness unrelated to vestibular dysfunction.

Patients need careful instruction about the potential side-effects of vestibular suppressants, particularly sedation, and how this may interfere with driving and operating machines. They should also know that treatment is symptomatic and intended for

Table 8.5 Pharmacological profile of commonly used vestibular suppressants

Generic name	Class	Action (antivertiginous/ antiemetic)	Sedation	Other side-effects
Cyclizine	Antihistaminic	AV+, AE+	+	Dry mouth
Diphenhydramine	Antihistaminic, anticholinergic	AV++, AE++	++	Dry mouth
Dimenhydrinate	Antihistaminic, anticholinergic	AV++, AE++	++	Dry mouth
Scopolamine	Anticholinergic	AV+, AE+++	+	Dry mouth, tachycardia, memory loss (elderly)
Cinnarizine	Calcium antagonist, antihistaminic	AV+	+	Weight gain, depression, parkinsonian syndrome
Diazepam	Benzodiazepine	AV++, AE+, anxiolytic	++	Lethargy, addiction, withdrawal symptoms
Lorazepam	Benzodiazepine	AV++, AE+, anxiolytic	++	Lethargy, addiction, withdrawal symptoms
Promethazine	Antihistaminic, anticholinergic, antidopaminergic	AV+++, AE+++	+++	Lethargy, dystonia, postural hypotension, dry mouth
Prochlorperazine	Antidopaminergic, antihistaminic	AV+, AE+++	++	Dystonia, postural hypotension, dry mouth
Metoclopramide	Antidopaminergic, anticholinergic	AE++	+	Dystonia, restlessness

AV = antivertiginous, AE = antiemetic

short-term application only. Some patients develop drug dependency, particularly with benzodiazepines but also with antihistamines such as dimenhydrinate.

Specific situations

Recovery from acute vestibular neuritis occurs spontaneously over days to weeks by central compensation. During the first 24–48 hours, when vertigo, nausea and vomiting are severe, patients need a potent vestibular suppressant and antiemetic (e.g. promethazine or dimenhydrinate). Thereafter, central compensation can be accelerated by vestibular rehabilitation (see page 169). In animal models, various drugs have been shown to promote central compensation (e.g. amphetamine, verapamil, caffeine and ginkgo) while others retard this process (e.g. dopamine antagonists, benzodiazepines, anticholinergics and antihistamines). In general, drugs that facilitate compensation are stimulants and drugs that inhibit compensation are sedatives. None of the accelerating substances, however, has proven its potential to promote central compensation from unilateral vestibular loss in a clinically significant way. However, evidence from a controlled trial suggests that steroids may increase the number of patients who recover peripheral function (see page 60). In patients with ill-compensated unilateral vestibular loss, antivertiginous drugs may alleviate symptoms to some extent, but their use is not advisable because of their interference with central compensation.

Motion sickness can be very distressing to susceptible individuals and is a good indication for vestibular suppressants. Meclizine, which is only mildly sedating, can be tried first. When symptoms are severe, dimenhydrinate is preferable. Transdermal scopolamine is also very effective but works only when applied well in advance, so the patch has to be put in place a few hours before embarking on a journey. *Mal de debarquement* designates the persistent sensation of movement after returning from a boat trip. It is not associated with nausea and usually ceases after several hours or a few days. Pharmacological intervention is not effective.

Recurrent vertigo of unknown cause (benign recurrent vertigo) is a common diagnosis, even in specialised neuro-otologic clinics after full investigation. When the term *benign recurrent vertigo* is used a link to migraine is commonly implicated (see page 78). Whether patients are actually suffering from vestibular migraine, Ménière's disease or vestibular paroxysmia may become evident later in the course of the disease. For symptomatic treatment one should prescribe vestibular suppressants, preferably suppositories or buccal tablets, for self-administration during prolonged and severe attacks. For prophylaxis one may try low-dose carbamazepine when attacks last in the order of seconds and recur frequently, assuming that neurovascular compression (see page 86) could be the underlying mechanism (or just knowing that brief attacks of vertigo often respond to carbamazepine, no matter what the cause is). When attacks last longer than seconds, migraine prophylaxis can be tried, such as with a beta-blocker or flunarizine (see page 78). Alternatively, one may suspect early Ménière's disease, even in the absence of aural symptoms, and try betahistine (although with a low probability of an effect, even if it is Ménière's disease). Finally, if all this has failed, it can be justified to try a non-sedating dose of a vestibular suppressant for long-term prophylaxis.

Ten common vestibular suppressants and antiemetics
Note that nomenclature and availability may vary between countries.

Cyclizine
- *Pharmacology:* Piperazine with antihistaminic and anticholinergic properties. Peak efficacy two to six hours after ingestion.
- *Indication:* Vertigo of mild to moderate severity; motion sickness (should be taken one hour in advance).
- *Side-effects:* Less sedation than other vestibular suppressants. Dry mouth and other anticholinergic effects.
- *Dose:* 50 mg orally, IV or intramuscularly; maximum 150 mg/d.

Diphenhydramine

- *Pharmacology:* H_1-receptor antagonist with antihistaminic and anticholinergic action. Half-life four to six hours.
- *Indication:* Vertigo and nausea of moderate severity; motion sickness.
- *Side-effects:* Moderate sedation, dry mouth. May exacerbate glaucoma, urinary retention and asthma.
- *Dose:* 25–50 mg orally or 50 mg rectally, every six to eight hours.

Dimenhydrinate

- *Pharmacology:* Dimenhydrinate is the theoclate salt of diphenhydramine (see previous entry) and has very similar pharmacological properties.
- *Indication:* Vertigo and nausea of moderate severity; motion sickness.
- *Side-effects:* Moderate sedation, dry mouth. May exacerbate glaucoma, urinary retention and asthma.
- *Dose:* 50–100 mg orally or 150 mg rectally, every six to eight hours.

Scopolamine

- *Pharmacology:* Muscarin receptor antagonist (anticholinergic), delivered by a transdermal system (patch). Powerful antiemetic effect.
- *Indication:* Prophylaxis for motion sickness; not effective when applied during acute motion sickness.
- *Side-effects:* Mild sedation, dry mouth, memory loss and hallucinations (particularly in elderly people), tachycardia, exacerbation of urinary retention and glaucoma. Withdrawal symptoms (nausea, imbalance, headaches) may develop when used for more than three days.
- *Dose:* Patch contains 1.5 mg scopolamine and releases 0.5 mg within three days. To be applied behind the ear six hours before embarking.

Cinnarizine

- *Pharmacology:* Calcium antagonist and antihistaminic action with antivertiginous effects. Half-life three to six hours.
- *Indication:* Acute vertigo of mild to moderate severity; also effective for motion sickness.
- *Side-effects:* Only minor sedation, but weight gain, depression and a reversible parkinsonian syndrome can be a problem.
- *Dose:* 75 mg every eight hours.

Diazepam

- *Pharmacology:* Benzodiazepine (GABA agonist). Half-life 24–48 hours, maximum effect two hours after oral intake, immediate effect after intravenous (IV) administration.
- *Indication:* Acute vertigo and nausea, particularly when sedation and anxiolytic effect is also desired. Less potent antiemetic than diphenhydramine, dimenhydrinate and promethazine. Low doses can be used for one to four weeks in patients with anxiety-related dizziness.
- *Side-effects:* Drowsiness, lethargy, increased risk of falls, dependency, withdrawal symptoms (nervousness, anxiety, sleep disturbances, seizures). Intravenous

application may cause apnoea and cardiac arrest, especially in patients with pulmonary disease.

- *Dose:* 2–10 mg orally, rectally or IV every six hours.

Lorazepam

- *Pharmacology:* Benzodiazepine (GABA agonist). Half-life 9–19 hours, maximum effect two hours after oral intake, immediate effect after IV or buccal administration. Accumulates less than diazepam due to shorter half-life and lack of active metabolites (the same holds true for clonazepam).
- *Indication:* Acute vertigo and nausea, particularly when sedation and anxiolytic effect is also desired. Low doses can be used for one to four weeks in patients with anxiety-related dizziness.
- *Side-effects:* Drowsiness, lethargy, increased risk of falls, dependency, withdrawal symptoms (nervousness, anxiety, sleep disturbances, seizures). Intravenous application may cause apnoea and cardiac arrest, especially in patients with pulmonary disease.
- *Dose:* 0.5–2 mg orally, IV or into muscle, every eight hours or 3–6 mg buccally every eight hours.

Promethazine

- *Pharmacology:* Phenothiazine with mostly antihistaminic action, but also anticholinergic and antidopaminergic properties. Half-life 16–19 hours.
- *Indication:* Acute vertigo with severe nausea and vomiting, when additional sedation is acceptable.
- *Side-effects:* Sedation, dry mouth, blurred vision, orthostatic hypotension, rarely dystonia or parkinsonian symptoms.
- *Dose:* 25 mg orally or into muscle, every eight hours. Caution! Intravenous application may cause tissue damage including gangrene.

Prochlorperazine

- *Pharmacology:* Phenothiazine, antidopaminergic agent with additional antihistaminic and anticholinergic properties. Main effect is antiemetic by blocking of dopaminergic transmission in the chemoreceptor trigger zone. Half-life 10 hours.
- *Indication:* Nausea and vomiting.
- *Side-effects:* Moderate sedation, dystonia, parkinsonian symptoms, akathisia, orthostatic hypotension, dry mouth, blurred vision. May exacerbate glaucoma and urinary retention. Elderly patients more susceptible to side-effects.
- *Dose:* 10 mg orally or into muscle every 6 hours or 25 mg rectally every 12 hours or 3 to 6 mg buccally.

Metoclopramide

- *Pharmacology:* D_2-receptor antagonist at the chemoreceptor trigger zone with additional anticholinergic effects and prokinetic action in the gastrointestinal tract. No effect on vestibular vertigo or motion sickness. Can be used in combination with vestibular suppressants. Rapid onset of action after 30–60 minutes. Half-life three to six hours.
- *Indication:* Nausea and vomiting.

- *Side-effects:* Dystonia, particularly in children, restlessness, drowsiness, fatigue, lethargy. parkinsonian symptoms and tardive dyskinesia with long-term use.
- *Dose:* 5–10 mg orally every 8 hours, or 20 mg rectally every 8–12 hours, or 10–20 mg IV.

Surgical treatment of vertigo

Surgery is only rarely required in vertiginous patients. When surgery is considered in patients with vertigo, the final decision should be made by a neuro-otologist. To minimise the risk, the operation should be performed by a dedicated ear surgeon.

Selective vestibular neurectomy is a routine procedure for removal of acoustic neuromas, but for treatment of refractory Ménière's disease it has been widely replaced by intratympanic gentamicin. Endolymphatic sac surgery for Ménière's disease also appears obsolete after a controlled trial has shown that it is no more effective than a sham operation. Very few patients with BPPV are refractory to conservative treatment with positional manoeuvres (less than 0.5% in our experience) and may require plugging of the posterior canal. This is achieved by drilling through the mastoid, opening the perilymphatic space of the canal and packing it with bone dust. Similarly rare are patients with refractory vestibular paroxysmia and a clear-cut vascular nerve compression on MRI allowing identification of the affected side. These patients may profit from surgical decompression of the nerve. Once in their lifetime neurologists or ENT surgeons may come across a patient with superior canal dehiscence who needs surgical repair of the bony roof of the affected canal.

Evidence-based treatment

Neuro-otology is a late starter when it comes to scientific assessment of treatment efficacy. Only a few randomised trials of sufficient size and rigor have been conducted. Table 8.6 lists the evidence for various treatments of vestibular disorders according to systematic reviews

Table 8.6 Evidence for treatments of dizziness and vertigo (from the Cochrane Library, October 2015)

Disorder	Intervention	Evidence for efficacy
Vestibular neuritis	Steroids	lacking
Acute and chronic unilateral vestibulopathy	Vestibular rehabilitation	moderate/strong
Bilateral vestibulopathy	Vestibular rehabilitation	moderate*
BPPV (posterior canal)	Epley's manoeuvre	strong
	Semont's manoeuvre	moderate
Ménière's disease	Low salt diet/diuretics	lacking
	Betahistine	lacking
	Intratympanic steroids	moderate
	Intratympanic gentamicin	moderate
	Endolymphatic sac surgery	lacking

* Based on a non-Cochrane systematic review

of randomised trials by the Cochrane Collaboration (for current updates see: www.cochrane.org). Properly conducted trials are largely lacking for treatment of other common vestibular disorders such as vestibular migraine, orthostatic dizziness and persistent perceptual dizziness. This may look like a sad state of affairs at the end of this book but it can be equally seen as a huge research opportunity for any young doctor diving into the vestibular world!

Further reading

Books

Baloh RW, Halmagyi GM (eds.). *Disorders of the Vestibular System.* Oxford: Oxford University Press, 1996.

Baloh RW, Kerber K. *Baloh and Honrubia's Clinical Neurophysiology of the Vestibular System.* New York: Oxford University Press, 2010.

Brandt T, Dieterich M, Strupp M. *Vertigo and Dizziness: Common Complaints.* London: Springer, 2013.

Bronstein AM (ed.). *Vertigo and Imbalance.* Oxford: Oxford University Press, 2013.

Eggers S, Zee D (eds.). *Vertigo and Imbalance: Clinical Neurophysiology of the Vestibular System. Handbook of Clinical Neurophysiology,* vol. 9. Amsterdam: Elsevier, 2010.

Furman JM, Cass SP, Whitney SL. *Vestibular Disorders: A Case Study Approach.* New York: Oxford University Press, 2010.

Harris, JP, Nguyen QT (eds.). *Meniere's Disease. Otolaryngologic Clinics of North America,* vol. 43, 2010.

Herdman SJ, Clendaniel PT. *Vestibular Rehabilitation.* Philadelphia: F. A. Davis, 2014.

Kaga K. *Vertigo and Balance Disorders in Children.* New York: Springer, 2014.

Leigh RJ, Zee DS. *The Neurology of Eye Movements.* New York: Oxford University Press, 2015.

Jacobson GP, Shepard N. *Balance Function Assessment and Management.* San Diego: Plural Publishing, 2014.

Articles

Brandt T, Huppert D. Fear of heights and visual height intolerance. *Curr Opin Neurol* 2014; 27: 111–7.

Bronstein AM, Golding JF, Gresty MA. Vertigo and dizziness from environmental motion: visual vertigo, motion sickness, and drivers' disorientation. *Semin Neurol* 2013; 33: 219–30.

Bronstein AM, Pavlou M. Balance. *Handb Clin Neurol* 2013; 110: 189–208.

Cha YH, Lee H, Santell LS, Baloh RW. Association of benign recurrent vertigo and migraine in 208 patients. *Cephalalgia* 2009; 29: 550–5.

Curthoys IS, Halmagyi GM. Vestibular compensation: a review of the oculomotor, neural and clinical consequences of unilateral vestibular loss. *J Vestib Res* 1995; 5: 67–107.

Fife TD, Iverson DJ, Lempert T, et al. Quality Standards Subcommittee, American Academy of Neurology. Practice parameter: therapies for benign paroxysmal positional vertigo (an evidence-based review). *Neurology* 2008; 70: 2067–74.

Grad A, Baloh RW. Vertigo of vascular origin: clinical and electronystagmographic features in 84 cases. *Arch Neurol* 1989; 46: 281–4.

Headache Classification Committee of the International Headache Society (IHS). *International Classification of Headache Disorders,* 3rd edition (beta version). www.ihs-classification.org/_downloads/ mixed/International-Headache-Classification-III-ICHD-III-2013-Beta.pdf.

Hoppe LJ, Ipser J, Gorman JM, Stein DJ. Panic disorder. *Handb Clin Neurol* 2012; 106: 363–74.

Hüfner K, Barresi D, Glaser M et al. Vestibular paroxysmia. *Neurology* 2008; 71: 1006–14.

Kattah JC, Talkad AV, Wang DZ, Hsieh YH, Newman-Toker DE. HINTS to diagnose stroke in the acute vestibular syndrome: three-step bedside oculomotor examination more sensitive than early MRI diffusion-weighted imaging. *Stroke* 2009; 40: 3504–10.

Kim S, Oh YM, Koo JW, Kim JS. Bilateral vestibulopathy: clinical characteristics and diagnostic criteria. *Otol Neurotol* 2011; 32: 812–7.

Lee H, Sohn SI, Cho YW, et al. Cerebellar infarction presenting isolated vertigo: frequency and vascular topographical patterns. *Neurology* 2006; 67: 1178–83.

Lempert T, Brandt T, Dieterich M, Huppert D. How to identify psychogenic disorders of stance and gait: a video study in 37 patients. *J Neurol* 1991; **238**: 140–6.

Lempert T, Olesen J, Furman J, et al. Vestibular migraine: diagnostic criteria. *J Vest Res* 2012; **22**: 167–2.

Lopez L, Bronstein AM, Gresty MA, Rudge P, du Boulay E. Torsional nystagmus: a neuro-otological and MRI study of thirty-five cases. *Brain* 1992; **115**: 1107–21.

Matsuoka AJ, Harris JP. Autoimmune inner-ear disease: a retrospective review of forty-seven patients. *Audiol Neuro-otol* 2013; **18**: 228–39.

Moya A, Sutton R, Ammirati F et al. Task force for the diagnosis and management of syncope. Guidelines for the diagnosis and management of syncope. *Eur Heart J* 2009; **30**: 2631–71.

Murdin L, Schilder AG. Epidemiology of balance symptoms and disorders in the community: a systematic review. *Otol Neurotol* 2015; **36**: 387–92.

Ong AC, Myint PK, Shepstone L, Potter JF. A systematic review of the pharmacological management of orthostatic hypotension. *Int J Clin Pract* 2013; **67**: 633–46.

Parnes LS, McClure JA. Free floating endolymph particles: a new operative finding during posterior semicircular canal occlusion. *Laryngoscope* 1992; **102**: 988–92.

Staab JP. Chronic subjective dizziness. *Continuum* 2012; **18**: 1118–41.

Strupp M, Arbusov V, Maag KP, Gall C, Brandt T. Vestibular exercises improve central vestibulo-spinal compensation after vestibular neuritis. *Neurology* 1998; **51**: 838–44.

Media for patients

Dizziness and Balance Problems: www.brainandspine.org.uk.

Vestibular Disorders Association: www.vestibular.org.

Meniere Man. The Self Help Book for Meniere's Vertigo. New York: Page Addie Press 2013.

Ménière's Society: www.menieres.org.uk.

Poe D. *The Consumer Handbook on Dizziness and Vertigo*. Sedona: Auricle Ink Publ., 2005.

Vestibular Migraine Forum: www.mvertigo.org.

Wilcox E. *Benign Positional Vertigo: An Essential Guide to Coping with and Treating BPPV*. Kindle edition, 2015.

Index